Sudden Infant Death Syndrome

Learning from stories about SIDS, motherhood and loss

Dawne J Gurbutt

Radcliffe Publishing
Oxford • Seattle

Radcliffe Publishing Ltd
18 Marcham Road
Abingdon
Oxon OX14 1AA
United Kingdom

www.radcliffe-oxford.com
Electronic catalogue and worldwide online ordering facility.

British Library Cataloguing in Publication Data

A catalogue record for this book is available from the British Library.

ISBN-10 1 84619 038 X
ISBN-13 978 1 84619 038 4

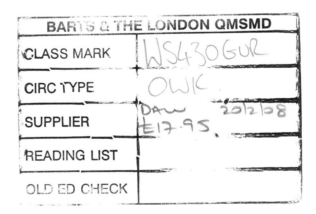
Typeset by Anne Joshua & Associates, Oxford
Printed and bound by TJI Digital, Padstow, Cornwall

'. . . a cry of anguish is heard in Ramah – mourning and weeping unrestrained. Rachel weeps for her children, refusing to be comforted – for her children are dead.'

Jeremiah 31.15

For Jessica and Tom

Contents

Preface

Much has been written about sudden infant death syndrome (SIDS), sometimes known as 'cot death'; many research projects have studied potential causes and sought to identify risk factors. Yet still much remains unknown about what causes an apparently healthy baby to die suddenly, unexpectedly and without an ascertainable cause.

The research for this study formed part of a larger pathological study into sudden infant death syndrome. I met and interviewed women who had recently experienced SIDS, and professionals and volunteers (some of whom had also experienced SIDS) who sought to try and offer support to these newly bereaved mothers. I met members of support groups and reviewed the literature made available to mothers whose infants had died. Although I did meet some fathers and grandparents, I mainly met mothers and so this book reflects primarily conversations with mothers relatively soon after their babies had died. This is a book primarily about SIDS, but also about maternal grief – from ancient times when writers have sought to express the depth of grief they have alluded to maternal grief following the death of a child.

It is hard to know sometimes where to start, what to keep in and what to leave out. I have tried to order these comments in some way to give them structure, and in doing so, some element of selection occurs. I have tried to represent as accurately as I can the essence of what they told me and to be careful in conveying the meaning as well as just using actual words. I was particularly concerned about anonymity and confidentiality and this necessitated leaving some things out and altering some details where appropriate.

Although I had previously worked for a lengthy time in practice before engaging with this research, I found the space to reflect on

SIDS and the way practitioners respond to SIDS a learning experience. This book has been written primarily to enable others to reflect on some of the stories which circulate around SIDS. They are not always easy stories to write or easy stories to read – but they are stories that need to be told and heard so that we can increase understanding of SIDS.

Dawn Gurbutt
November 2006

Acknowledgements

I would like to thank all the women who allowed themselves to be interviewed for my research study and all those who supported me in and contributed in any way to my research. I would also like to thank friends and colleagues who encouraged me to write a text and especially Gill Nineham for encouraging me to write *this* book in this way – I hope the end product approaches what you envisaged.

I especially want to thank Russell – who always believes that I will be able to do the things that I find daunting – for his continual support, encouragement and practical help. We have made a good team. Thanks too to my children who constantly teach me so much about life and love – and are inspiring company. Finally, thanks to my mother-in-law Sheila, who many years ago shared her particular story of motherhood with me.

About the author

Dawne Gurbutt has a keen interest in narratives and qualitative research. She has been engaged in a number of projects exploring different aspects of women's lives. Her career has included nursing, midwifery and health visiting. She worked in community practice for over a decade in the North of England, prior to working in the university sector. Her HEI work has included teaching, research, management and consultancy. She is married with two children.

Abbreviations

BtoS   Back to Sleep campaign
CESDI Confidential Enquiry into Sudden Deaths in Infancy
CONI   Care of Next Infant programme
GP   General practitioner
SIDS   Sudden infant death syndrome

Chapter 1

What's the story? Understanding narratives

We are all storied

We all know about stories. Stories are part of every culture and part of all of our lives. We are surrounded by stories of one kind or another: newspapers, conversations, fiction and drama. We are all engaged in telling and listening to stories, weaving our experiences into words. Some of our earliest memories may be of listening to the stories our mothers told us. Those stories had a shape, a beginning, middle and an end. Through them we learned to shape our world – to look for beginnings and to recognise endings. We learned about characters and the importance of events. At primary school we learned to write our lives in stories – to select events out of all the things that were happening to us and to give them a shape and a form, to try to find a place to begin and to decide where to end. We learned to communicate something of ourselves in that form – to describe our lives as a series of episodes. We learned to orally put together our autobiography – events, thoughts and emotions – in a way that could be shared with other people. And then as we learned the art of telling our stories, of engaging other people in our lives, storytelling became a part of what we are, how we live and how we make sense of our complicated and confusing world.[1]

We constantly tell stories, from sharing the events of our day to sharing the circumstances and contexts that we believe have shaped our human experience and personalities. We are encouraged to tell the story of who we are and what has happened to us in a variety of settings, from meeting people who have newly entered our lives, to sharing something of ourselves with strangers, to recounting how we developed our current skills in a job interview, to explaining our actions to our children and friends, or explaining events to ourselves in our diaries. We constantly tell stories; they are part of the fabric and currency of our lives. Some of the stories we only tell once, some we tell over and over again. Some stories are instantly forgotten in the plethora of new stories that are developing around us, and some are frequently revisited and often retold, and may be re-shaped by subsequent events, constant reminders of the integral themes of our lives. We choose our words and we select our audiences.

Some of our stories may not seem significant to other people, but they are highly significant to us and to those closest to us. My teenagers still like to hear particular stories about things they did as small children. The events I recount are incredibly familiar; they are tales that have been told and retold, but they still enjoy the story. Part of the appeal is in the telling; they are waiting for the elements that they are familiar with; the triggers to which they can respond. But part of their enjoyment in the story is the link with the past, with the people they were and are. These narratives locate them within a wider discourse, relate them to significant others in their lives, and remind them that they are part of a wider network. The stories tell of events that have shaped their identities. They are also stories about relationship. As a mother, when I tell them stories about their childhood, I am also telling stories about my mothering – about the things that I remember because they were funny, or touching or sad – but things which reaffirm our relationship. I am telling them 'our' history. Nor does it stop there – I tell them the stories my grandparents, parents and in-laws have told me. I am the repository of parts of a family history – and so we connect the past with the present – the living with the dead. Whilst I am alive, some of their stories of love, romance, bravery and adventure will persist, and we will all have a sense of the people they were and are; how their qualities, their lives and their legacy of stories have shaped our own lives. Their history sets us wondering about ourselves, our strengths and weaknesses, potential latent talents and capabilities, and enables our imagining of what other stories could have been told if things had been different.

In the autumn of 2004, I was visiting a museum with my father and children that offered the opportunity to trace family members killed in the Great War of 1914–1918. My father had often shared with me the story of his uncle's death at the close of the 'war to end all wars' and the effect that it had on his grandparents. The story he shared was situated in the family grief experience and his grandmother's reaction to that great and significant loss. This was a grief that was mirrored a million times in the experience of families like ours, as that conflict played itself out across Europe. So there we were, putting details into a computer with an expectation of finding out the 'facts' that would validate and confirm the story we knew. We found 'Uncle Bill', but we also uncovered some discrepancies in dates and locations (perhaps due in part to the logistics of transferring information in those years and the scale of the task). But we also found where he was buried and details of the attack in which he died. A slightly different story in its detail to the one we knew, but a recognisable one and one which re-connected us with our history.[2] In the summer of 2005, I travelled with my own family to Belgium, to Flanders Fields, and searched for his grave. In a field of a thousand graves, after a long search, we found 'him'. In the commonwealth cemeteries, all the graves appear the same and yet each is different for the families whose relatives are buried there. I couldn't take my eyes off that family headstone. Here was my ancestor, a young man with the same name as my father, buried with his comrades in a foreign field. The stories I knew of his life, the legacy of his name passing to my father and other young men of the next generation came back to me. Standing in the Belgian sunshine, in a peaceful place that belies its own violent history, I shared those stories with the next generation. I don't think any of us will forget that day, as historical facts learned in school became entwined with our story and the general became specific – here was someone we could relate to, a way for us to begin to try to understand. Why am I recalling this here, and why is that event significant? In part, because it is through stories and narratives that we live on in the memories of others and that we give meaning to our lives. Our identification with the stories of others offers us a way into understanding their experiences and making sense of who we are.

Stories, then, have a power beyond the words with which they are composed. It is important to look beyond and between the words and consider what is said and what is left unsaid. This process of unravelling meaning and uncovering information is part of the art of both storyteller and listener. The selection of beginnings and endings is part of defining who we are and of accepting that everything cannot always be told – so, the ordering and shaping of our stories becomes important.[3] Some stories are linear, with events seemingly occurring one after the other in sequence, and with responses to those events categorised and reflected upon. But other stories are a rich mixture of the told and the untold, the obvious and the hidden, the public and the private, the multiple threads of experience that tangle themselves together and give us some insights into the complexity of life.

Stories shape and are shaped by history, identity and relationships, as well as by the audience – the people who listen to the stories we tell. Stories are readily shaped by the listener; the questions they ask and the interest they show influence narratives. Other factors are important too, such as the time available to tell the story, and the rapport and confidence that exists between listener and story teller. So, in various ways, we *are* all storied, we tell stories, we listen to stories, we are part of the stories of others.

What's the story?

This is a book about stories. These were stories that mothers told and that I listened to as part of a research project;[4] stories told by mothers who had lived through a particular experience that had shaped and would continue to shape their lives. The term 'story' is often associated with fictional works. But I am using the term differently here. I want to describe some of the narratives of the women I interviewed. These were accounts of what had happened to them and their reactions to those happenings.

Teenagers sometimes ask 'What's the story?' as shorthand for asking what is happening, to find out some of the context to an event. This is closer to the meaning I am striving for here. Consider for a moment, the diversity and difference in the stories we tell in everyday life – the accounts of what has happened to us. Some are social chatter whilst others are explanatory and necessary for good communication; all tell the listener something about us, about our lives and about our ways of seeing the world. There are differences between stories that merely lay out the facts, and stories that offer interpretation, explanation and reflection. It becomes clear that stories are layered, embedded within one another; multifaceted and complex.

In research terms, the narratives I will refer to here have a context. These mothers did not approach me, I approached them. I told them what I was doing and invited them to participate. I already had a framework for their stories – I was going to ask them about their experiences in the context of sudden infant death syndrome (SIDS) and hopefully they would feel able to tell me about what had happened to them. It sounds straightforward and uncomplicated and at one level it is, but at another level it is also complex – how could they begin to put into words the enormity of what had happened in their lives? How could I ever, in an hour or two, gain a useful insight into all that had happened to them as mothers? The result is their stories, the beginnings and the ends to the particular accounts they shared with me (prompted in part by where I indicated they should begin by the way I framed my questions). They didn't all begin in the same place, they didn't all end their accounts in the same way, but there were patterns and similarities to the stories they told me. This is the stuff of which research is made: the patterns, the order, the continuities and discontinuities, the sameness and difference. These were the things maybe I was listening for, but in the process of listening I heard many different things. I learned so much more than I thought I would about SIDS, about identity, about mothers, about families and society, but mostly about maternal love and the immense, diabolical, indescribable, unfathomable pain that accompanies the loss of a child.

So what is the story? It is my account of listening to mothers talk about the loss of their child from SIDS, reading the accounts of

SIDS in newspapers, listening to the news broadcasts, and listening to parents in support groups talk about their experiences. The story is about SIDS and its impact on individuals and groups.

So, in this book I will refer to many stories. Some will be based on the comments of mothers, their 'stories', but alongside these I will also refer to other stories: in the newspapers and in government reports, and stories I read in books written by those who have experienced this sort of loss. There are also other narratives, those of other young mothers, of health professionals and volunteers who also told me stories about SIDS. These are stories I have woven together from what I have heard, not always as skilfully as I would have liked. They *are* stories about SIDS, but they are also stories about motherhood, about families, about life and death. However, I cannot capture here the silences, the tears, the textures, and the pain, the tangible and sometimes palpable sorrow of their loss. So, what is the story? It is multiple, fluid, dynamic and sometimes raw. Here it has a beginning and an end of sorts – that is the nature of the work of writing things down – but the real stories are bigger than this. They are bigger than words.

'You had to have been there'

I have always enjoyed working with people. I have always liked to engage with people and have, for a long time, made my living from talking and listening – and in some ways it is a skill of sorts – one which I still need to work on and perfect. But one of the consequences of my work as a talker and listener is that sometimes people tend to tell me things. Often at the start of my classes one of the students will share a story of something that has happened to them during the week, knowing that they will have a ready and appreciative audience. They are often tales of something amusing or absurd, often self-depreciating, and fairly often the story hinges on context – situational humour or an atmosphere that they find difficult to put into words. I am glad they try to find the words to share their experiences and together we often reach the point where I 'get' the story. Their stories are told with enthusiasm and obvious keenness to communicate what happened, and yet when they can't convey exactly what it was like they often resort to using the phrase 'perhaps you had to have been there'. It is a phrase that became very meaningful to me in my research.

The mothers I listened to transported me with their words to many of the places they had been – to the room where they went to attend to their infant and found their baby had died, to sitting in the Accident & Emergency department, to the funeral, to the graveside. I found this deeply moving and emotional; I was grateful to them for their honesty, for their capacity to share with me difficult and personal experiences. Their descriptions were often sensitive, graphic and compelling. But I have to acknowledge something very simple and yet profound: that I was not there. All I can pass on is what I recall from their accounts, from their stories. Therefore, it is important to acknowledge my role in shaping their stories as they are presented here – the questions I asked, the responses I gave, the emphasis I remember from what they said to me. The responsibility I feel is huge, as I want to be true to not only their words but also to their own meanings. This is the tension which exists for narrative researchers to seek to reproduce what they have heard in its true context, and avoid re-shaping or skewing what they have heard. But at the same time to recognise that the researcher is part of the story. I have tried my best, but the weight of responsibility lies heavily on me.[5]

What makes a story?

So, what are the stories that I have to tell about SIDS? There are good stories concerning the reduction in the number of SIDS deaths, and bad stories in which mothers were accused of involvement in the deaths of their infants. There are different viewpoints and perspectives embedded within and influencing each other. My research was carried out in 1999–2001. As part of the project, I interviewed a number of women whose infants had died of SIDS. These were the 'inside' stories of SIDS told by people who had lived through that experience. However, as already mentioned, there were other stories being told about SIDS at that time. There was a story in the newspapers concerning a woman in the same region whose children's deaths had originally been categorised as SIDS but were now being re-investigated as unlawful deaths.[6] This was a local story, a court case being played out in the region where I was working. The case captured a great deal of local as well as national media attention; it was relevant because it was regional and a case with 'human interest'. The story broke amidst a number of articles in the press that suggested that the classification of SIDS might be masking deaths due to unnatural causes.[7] It was suggested to me at the time that this was regarded by the media as a 'good' story. Yet, good for whom? Certainly not a good story for the mothers who were reading allegations made about a mother whose children had died of SIDS; not good for those who were working with families of children who had died of SIDS trying to provide support in the context of all the controversies surrounding SIDS in the newspapers. Throughout the period of my study there were other cases in the newspapers of other women whose infants had died and been classified as SIDS, and were now under suspicion and on trial following a second death in the family.[8] There were also the later appeals of some of these cases, and the acquittal of those women as some of the evidence used in court was questioned and found to be unreliable. Then there was the media coverage of the retention of the internal organs of infants and children at Alder Hey Hospital for research purposes. The organs had been kept, without parental consent, and in many cases had never been used for research purposes. It emerged that the doctor[9] at the centre of the organ retention scandal had a reputation for working with SIDS. Suddenly stories about SIDS were everywhere: stories that involved suspicion and accusation of mothers whose infants had died, SIDS as an unreliable category, and SIDS associated (indirectly) with poor research practices. These research practices had caused further pain and distress to grieving parents whose infants had died at Alder Hey Hospital. However misplaced the 'facts' of the associations between SIDS and Alder Hey might be, SIDS was in the news and for all the wrong reasons.

The accounts of SIDS that emerged at this time contrasted with more positive existing stories. References to the 'Back to Sleep' campaign (BtoS)[10] that emerged in 1991 were constantly in the media. This campaign had been publicised by the broadcaster Anne Diamond whose own son, Sebastian, had died of SIDS. BtoS encouraged parents to actively consider the sleeping position and environment of their babies. Parents were advised not to share their beds with their babies, and to ensure that their infants were placed down to sleep supine with their feet at the foot of the cot to avoid overheating. The campaign also encouraged parents to monitor the temperature of the bedroom and to avoid the use of high TOG-rated bedding. Attention was also drawn to the risks of smoking in the vicinity of young infants. BtoS became shorthand for a number of linked initiatives all concerned with the sleeping environment of the infant. As one health visitor put it:

> 'To say it was all about sleep position was to overlook a lot. There were all sorts of things which we were advising parents about.'

BtoS was credited with a substantial and sustained reduction in the number of deaths attributed to SIDS.[11]

In February 2000, the Confidential Enquiry into Sudden Deaths in Infancy (CESDI), commissioned by the NHS, commented on the impact of BtoS, and also highlighted the risks associated with smoking, as well as identifying other risk factors associated with SIDS, such as age and parity of the mother.[12]

It seemed as though references to SIDS were everywhere, in the media and in government reports. SIDS was visible through court cases, research reports and later in controversies relating to statistics used as evidence in court.[13] It seemed that SIDS was constantly in the news and there were both good and bad stories relating to SIDS. It is within this media and policy context that I interviewed women about their experiences of loss.

Times and places – situated stories

Occasionally you can be in a situation, perhaps at a party or a social gathering, where you are engaged in conversation and suddenly in the periphery of your consciousness you hear your own name mentioned. Suddenly, part of your focus is on what you were doing and part on straining to hear what is being said about you. These are comments that might not draw the attention of others, but are filtered out as important to you. So it is with SIDS, in the flood of information that was awash in the media at any given time – these mothers and those working with SIDS could see and hear information about SIDS everywhere and were tapping in to those constantly fluctuating streams of information. In addition, there was a plethora of writing and comment about grief that appears in the press every time there is an event that draws attention to the loss of life. This type of reporting includes articles outlining what grief is and guidance as to what 'normal' grief is like.[14] Add these elements together and you have a huge amount of suggestion, opinion and unsolicited guidance circulating around these mothers, as well as support. And in the midst of it all, the research project with which I was involved created an opportunity to listen to some mothers tell their stories of what it is actually like to experience SIDS.

My conversations with mothers about their experiences of SIDS took place as part of a wider research project searching for further insights into the causes of SIDS. The mothers who agreed to participate in the study were all interviewed between 6 weeks and 8 months of the deaths of their babies. Their words and comments are only a 'snapshot' of their experiences at a particular time and in a particular place. Over these months the different interviews took place at times when SIDS was 'in the news' to varying extents and with different emphasis. The women I interviewed and those I met through other contexts had to navigate and negotiate all sorts of information about SIDS, about grief and loss, and about motherhood. This included uncertainties about how to define and categorise SIDS,[15] and later disputes about the statistical calculation of the incidence and probability of SIDS within a single family. These uncertainties illustrated, for me, the complexities of SIDS. SIDS is a category of exclusion; therefore it is the classification that remains when all other causes of death have been ruled out. That is to say you cannot 'diagnose' SIDS, you can only identify that the death occurred without ascertainable cause and is therefore classified as SIDS. Therefore, uncertainties and instabilities around the classification of SIDS will always persist to some extent. This has a number of effects, not least that the cause of death can always be revisited as new information on potential causes of death emerges, and so there is no closure.[16]

It is important to remember that some of these accounts emerged as a result of research interviews, and this will have had some impact on the content of the sessions and the subsequent narratives. I saw each research participant once, and the interview was centred on their experiences of SIDS. Some of the women I interviewed commented that they found it beneficial to talk to someone outside of their situation – indeed some mothers related to me conversations they had had with strangers about their experiences. Although there were some similarities in the women's experiences, there were also differences. It is important to acknowledge that every experience is unique, but that there were some patterns that emerged. The interviews took place over a period of 2 years, and different media stories dominated the headlines at different times throughout that period. Media stories about SIDS formed a constantly changing backdrop to their accounts. There were other differences too: some women had other children and were engaged in supporting their families through the loss of a sibling as well as coping with their own grief. Some women had lost their only child and were aware of the potential loss of their identity as 'mothers'. Some women were pregnant again and others were hoping to have further children. Each situation is unique, individual and particular. These are not tidy stories with a clear ending. These are ongoing stories, the account of the start of a journey they did not choose to take and, although some reflected on what became similar landmarks, many still expressed how long a road was stretching before them.

Mediated stories

As I have already mentioned, stories do not happen in isolation and it is important to recognise and acknowledge the place of the listener, in this case myself as researcher, in formulating the stories that are explored here. As listeners, we constantly give out cues, show our interest and react in verbal and non-verbal ways. So it is important to reflect on the fact that these interviews took place at particular times and places and were, at least in part, a response to the situation we found ourselves in. My experiences as a health professional will have affected these interviews in some measure. I had experience of visiting people in their own homes.[17] In comparison to my previous experience as a health professional, the social texture of these interviews was notable. The majority of the interviews were conducted in a quiet atmosphere. Generally, on arrival, the mother would turn off the TV or radio – this seemed really important to me, as I had visited clients in their own homes for years and most of the time the TV or radio was a constant backdrop to any discussion. It seemed noteworthy that most of these interviews occurred without the distraction of this type of background noise. There were occasions when the TV or a video was on, as sometimes toddlers were present at the interviews and the TV was used by mothers to occupy them.

There were other factors too, as sometimes other family members or friends were present for all or part of the interviews supporting the mother. I wanted the women I met to feel as comfortable as possible. On one occasion a health visitor was present. All of these factors will have had an effect on what the mothers told me and maybe the way they described and talked about their experiences. The type of issues discussed may have been affected by my being a woman interviewing other women.[18] Much has been written about the way in which women interact with each other and the importance of gender in interviews. Most of the women I interviewed asked me if I had children of my own, and this may also have influenced how they spoke about their experiences. As a mother I felt that there was a common understanding of the child care services and the types of situations mothers of infant and young children find themselves in. I did ask questions about people's experiences, but also found that most of the mothers I interviewed told their stories with very few questions being asked.

The accounts they gave of their experiences were moving, thought provoking and honest. Sometimes there were tears and silences, sometimes their words flowed, and at other times the words seemed to tumble out seemingly unchecked. The interviews were not just about conversations either. I was sometimes invited to touch and smell things that had belonged to their babies or to look at photographs. For me, the experience of listening to these women's stories is beyond words; they were moments suspended in time, which were so meaningful that they will remain with me. They spoke of their love for their babies and the things they had found both helpful and unhelpful. I was very affected by these interviews. Reading the notes I made at the time can still move me to tears as I think about their loss and their willingness to talk to me about something so profound and life changing. Sometimes I felt very tearful as I left the house and reflected on the enormity of what they had told me. I felt the weight of the responsibility of having heard their stories. I hope when I write of these things I do justice to them and to their accounts of SIDS. Even now, a few years afterwards, I am aware that listening to their stories about SIDS has had a lasting effect on me. I am deeply appreciative of the opportunity to be a mother. I am constantly aware of how much we get wrong as a society and as healthcare professionals in dealing with bereavement. I am conscious of how suddenly ordinary days and ordinary events can be rendered extraordinary. And I am reminded of how important it is to care for and support people who have to face the unfaceable and just how large this figures in their stories when they *have* felt themselves to be supported.

There it is then, a mix of the good and the bad, personal stories, public stories, things which have helped, and things which have been less than useful and maybe even harmful. These are the stories that are the basis of this book. Personal and private stories set against the backdrop of multiple media stories and public information about grief and the process of grieving.

Continuing stories

Although, in writing this text, I have drawn on my research interviews with women whose infants had died of SIDS, I also attended sessions run by a support group for bereaved parents, talked to professionals working with SIDS, and studied a range of literature written for and made available to parents at times of bereavement.

Most of the accounts of grief on which this book is based were from a very early stage of bereavement. There is a possibility that the events that mothers describe may change in emphasis over time and that other landmarks may become increasingly important. It is crucial to recognise and acknowledge this and to note that, although elements of what has happened to us do not change, the way we describe them to others may alter over time for a whole variety of reasons.

Writing is always about trying to find a way of ordering things – of finding some way of determining a beginning, a place to start and this text is no exception. It is a real challenge to try to find a 'way in' to exploring some of the stories around SIDS, and there is always some degree of messiness involved in choosing a place to start. Always there are things that are lost in the telling simply because they do not easily fit into the stories we choose to tell and the narratives we construct. In trying to find a way to begin, I have stayed true to my metaphor of stories and have mapped out this book as a series of storytelling 'genres': so I begin with the love story of motherhood. This is the narrative of the maternal romance, of bonding with and nurturing a new infant, and the subsequent heartache which accompanies the loss. I have also explored the horror story – the media coverage of SIDS and the associations made between SIDS and unnatural deaths. I have considered the collection of short stories which are part of a journal – the public and private stories, the front stage and back-stage work of SIDS.[19] I have considered the infant's identity and the 'baby book': the words and pictures, places and spaces which define the infant's life. So, I have also included a chapter on picture books: the images which tell stories without requiring words. Finally I have considered the atlas of grief and SIDS – attempting in some way to map the experience from different perspectives and positions. In doing so, I acknowledge the episodic character of these stories, the elements of these stories which indicate that these stories are still incomplete and partial; there will be other stories still to be told – some relating to SIDS, some relating to learning to live with loss. This then is a small library of different perspectives and narratives, all of which tell particular stories about SIDS.

Notes and references

1 Academic texts refer to 'paradigms' or different ways of seeing the world. These might include different perspectives, but may also include different understandings of concepts or ways of interpreting information.
   Cresswell JW. *Qualitative Inquiry and Research Design; choosing among five traditions.* London: Sage; 1998.
   Haraway DJ. *Modest Witness@Second Millennium. FemaleMan Meets OncoMouse.* New York: Routledge; 1997.
   Foucault M. *The Birth of the Clinic: – an archaeology of medical perception.* London: Tavistock; 1973.
2 Walter T. *The Revival of Death.* London: Routledge; 1999.
   This gives an explanation of how one 'story' can be multiple depending on the context and location. Stories are not generally linear and ordered, but are located within particular settings and may be viewed differently from different perspectives and by different people. The example is used of the competing accounts or versions of the death of a soldier in the Great War, and how these varying accounts all come to be compared and contrasted.
3 It was interesting for me to note the general quietness of the homes during the interviews (except for the presence of toddlers and the occasional interruption of the doorbell or telephone). This is sometimes referred to as the 'social texture' of interviews. I particularly noticed that women spontaneously turned off the television prior to being interviewed, and gave their full attention to talking about their experiences. This was in sharp contrast to my years of experience as a home visitor when the drone of daytime television was a constant backdrop to visits and discussions. The quiet ambience of these home interviews was notable.
4 The nature of the research project is outlined later in the chapter.
5 Skeggs (1995) comments: '*Thinking through issues of ethnographic representation raises many more ethical issues and confronts the power relations involved in research. When writing about the thoughts and actions of others you have to think about what you are doing with their words and how you are using your descriptions of their actions.*'
   Skeggs B, editor. *Feminist Cultural Theory Process and Production.* Manchester: Manchester University Press; 1995.
6 For an account of Sally Clark's experience see:
   Batt J. *Stolen Innocence.* London: Edbury Press; 2004.
7 The 'Think Dirty' campaign was also reported in the news. Green (1999) cited an Australian investigative protocol which advised practitioners to '*Think Dirty*' when presented with a sudden unexpected infant death. He also commented, '. . . *if we assumed that the*

numbers of adults who harm their children have remained fairly constant over the years, then in the relatively low number of baby deaths currently occurring the proportion of 'suspicious deaths' is increased accordingly. It follows that all of us involved in such deaths should approach them with suspicion, albeit cautiously expressed.'
Green MA. Time to put cot death to bed? *BMJ.* 1999; **319**: 697–8.

8 See the Angela Canning case. Her first child's death was categorised as SIDS but was reinvestigated when her second child died. She was acquitted in 2003.

9 Dick van Veltzen was a Dutch researcher working at Alder Hey Hospital, Liverpool, during the period it emerged that Alder Hey Hospital had retained children's organs at post mortem without parental consent. It was reported that Van Veltzen had a research profile that included research into SIDS.

10 The Back to Sleep campaign (1991) was part of a Foundation for the Study of Infant Death (FSID) initiative to reduce the incidence of SIDS by advising parents about sleep position and maintenance of infant body temperature.
Foundation for the Study of Infant Death. *Reduce the Risk 'Back to Sleep'.* London: FSID; 1991.

11 Fleming P, Blair P, Bacon C, Berry J, editors. *Sudden Unexpected Deaths in Infancy: the CESDI SUDI studies 1993–1996.* London: The Stationery Office; 2000.
This enquiry report was edited by Peter Fleming, with a foreword by Professor Roy Meadow.

12 For an exploration of risk factors associated with SIDS see CESDI reports, (reviewed quinquennially), and also the FSID website www.sids.org.uk/fsid/ (accessed 18 September 2006).

13 As in the evidence given by Professor Meadow, an expert witness but not a medical statistician, in the Sally Clark trial, 1999. This statistical evidence was later scrutinised and identified as containing inaccuracies. Meadow later faced a GMC investigation.

14 Such articles often appear in the press as 'comment' to accompany breaking news about a tragedy or disaster involving loss of life. Usually based on models of bereavement, such pieces offer an 'insight' into the grief experience – often referring to 'stages of grief' (e.g. Thomas Stuttaford, columnist for *The Times*).

15 Emery JL, Waite AJ. Debate on cot death. These deaths must be prevented without victimising parents. *BMJ.* 2000; **320**: 310.
Bacon C. Introduction. In: Fleming P, Blair P, Bacon C, Berry J, editors. *Sudden Unexpected Deaths in Infancy: the CESDI SUDI studies 1993–1996.* London: The Stationery Office; 2000.
Green MA. Time to put cot death to bed? *BMJ.* 1999; **319**: 697–8.
Limerick S. Not time to put cot death to bed. *BMJ.* 1999; **319**: 698–700.

See the above references for consideration of some of the difficulties in categorising SIDS, including whether utilising the SIDS category can 'mask' other causes of death.

For international differences in using the SIDS classification, see:

Rambaud C, Guilleminault C, Campbell P. Definition of the sudden infant death syndrome. *BMJ.* 1994; **308**: 1439.

For relevant SIDS studies, see:

Bacon CJ. Cot death after CESDI. *Arch Dis Child.* 1997; **76**(2): 171–3.

Blair PS. Smoking and sudden infant death syndrome. *Food Chem Toxicol.* 1996; **34**(11): 1195.

Blair PS, Fleming PJ, Leach CEA *et al.* A clinical comparison of SIDS and explained sudden infant deaths: how healthy and how normal. *Arch Dis Child.* 2000; **82**(2): 98–106.

Carpentier RG, Gardner A, Pursall E, McWeeny PM, Emery JL. Identification of some infants at immediate risk of dying unexpectedly and justifying intensive study. *Lancet.* 1979; **2**(8138): 343–6.

16 'Closure' is a term utilised by psychologists and others to indicate that the individual involved is able to draw a line under elements of an experience and begin to come to terms with their current situation. The fact that SIDS can be revisited at any time, and the publicity generated by the Clark (1999) and Canning (2002) cases, meant that mothers I interviewed were aware that they were unlikely to achieve 'closure' in relation to the cause of death.

17 I had previously worked in community practice as a registered practitioner for 11 years.

18 For comment on utilising feminist methodology and approaches see:

Haraway DJ. *Modest Witness@Second Millennium. FemaleMan Meets OncoMouse.* New York: Routledge; 1997.

Oakley A. Gender methodology and people's ways of knowing: some problems with feminism and the paradigm debate in social science. *Sociology.* 1998; **32**(4): 707–31.

Oakley A. *Experiments in Knowing: Gender and method in the social sciences.* Cambridge: Polity Press; 2000.

Stanley L, Wise S. Method, methodology and epistemology in feminist research processes. In: Wise L, editor. *Feminist Praxis Research, Theory and Epistemology in Feminist Sociology.* London: Routledge; 1990.

For practical reflections on women and data collection see:

Gurbutt DJ, Gurbutt R. The effect of gender on data collection with nurses who work with women in the community. *Community Pract.* 2001; **75**(7): 253-5.

19 Goffman E. *The Presentation of Self in Everyday Life.* Harmondsworth: Penguin; 1979.

Chapter 2

The love story

The love story is part of the culture of Europe, the overwhelming love for another person, which proves itself to be life changing in one way or another and is a frequently used genre familiar to many readers. It is a captivating and compelling story. In this chapter I will consider the way mothers described how they felt about their infants, the sudden loss of their babies, and how they continued to express their love for their babies.

The central motif of the love story, the intertwining of one's life with another person and the subsequent insights into their personality and identity, has been used by authors and researchers writing about bereavement. Hallam, Hockey & Howarth (1999)[1] describe the way a widow's identity is caught up in that of her husband and how she may feel herself, following bereavement, to be only a part of the person she once felt herself to be. Jane Littlewood (2001) likens the bereavement of a widow to a 'harlequin romance' referring to the story in which Harlequin is reported to be invisible to everyone but his faithful Columbine.[2] She uses this story to explore the experience of bereavement and the way in which the bereaved person has a continued, reciprocal relationship with the person who has died. This is a relationship which is meaningful and persists within its context despite the fact that it is invisible to other people. Hallam, Hockey & Howarth[1] also trace the many and multiple ways in which relationships continue after a death; this is discussed more fully in a later chapter. This sense of having lost part of oneself is a recurrent theme in bereavement literature; these descriptions trace a continued love story that impacts and shapes the life of the surviving partner.

Women who have written about the loss of their children also describe their continued relationship with, and love for, the child who has died. Pam Elder (1998), writing about the loss of her daughter Kate, a university student, describes vividly her continued love for her child and the way that she feels Kate's presence to such an extent that she feels people who get to know her, also come to know Kate. When I first read Pam Elder's chapter on the sudden loss of Kate, I was much moved.[3] Here was a family writing about a love story, their love story – of a daughter and sister, who remains a part of their lives. Even now, months on from my first reading of her work, her account, for its rawness and honesty, is still highly evocative and emotional to read – for this is the stuff of which love stories are made. There are many other published accounts of maternal love.[4]

This chapter is concerned with the experiences of a group of women whose babies had died of SIDS. Much has been written about maternal love and the mother–child bond. In the West, due to the relative wealth of society, the dominance of the biomedical model and its associated medical interventions and other social factors, there is a general expectation that parents will not outlive their children. So, for a parent to experience the death of a child places them immediately into a small group whose experiences are 'other'[5] to those of the majority. But this is compounded in SIDS by the sudden and unanticipated loss of an apparently healthy infant without 'ascertainable cause'.[6] The loss of the infant is rendered even more traumatic by the fact that the baby was usually well and showed no sign of an impending problem, leaving parents to question whether they have missed something significant.[7]

This chapter explores the ongoing love story of mothering, albeit interrupted by the infant's sudden death. It will also focus on how the bereaved parents in this study represented their infant to other people and spoke about their baby. At the same time it is necessary to acknowledge that talking about their babies is part of the experience of being a new mother, and is not in itself a practice that is unusual. It is also important to recognise the particular characteristics of SIDS and their effect on the maternal love story. The mothers in this study often described a pattern of events that separated them from their infants at a time when, in other contexts, parents would be encouraged to be with their child.[8] I will also consider the ways in which these mothers made their ongoing relationship with their infants visible via the funeral, objects and the infants' graves.

Representing the infant

Most mothers would acknowledge that motherhood brings with it large changes in lifestyle, role and identity. Some of these effects are physical, some are emotional, and others social, but all bring about a significant shift in identity. Acquiring the primary responsibility for the nurture and nutrition of a young infant necessitates a reappraisal of roles and responsibilities. Western society firmly places the responsibility for care of infants on their mothers. In spite of the media emphasis given to the emergence of the capable 'new man', it is still the case that many of the day-to-day practical tasks relating to the care of a new baby are generally, although not always, assigned to the mother. Hence, although fatherhood alters identity too, it is the mother who often adopts the identity of the primary carer. Much has been written about the importance of the process of bonding or attachment that takes place between the mother and infant in the early stages of the infant's life.[9] Lack of a secure attachment is seen as problematic for both mother and child and is often viewed as symptomatic of deeper concerns. Generally the bond of affection between mother and child is viewed as a strong and unshakeable attachment. It is this generation of love that is fundamental to understanding the love stories associated with infants who have died of SIDS.

Most of the mothers I interviewed spontaneously mentioned their relationship with their baby. Some described their baby as the fulfilment of their desire to be mothers:

'I longed to be mother . . . he was so special.'

Others commented on their babies as 'much wanted' or recalled:

> 'I was looking forward so much to the birth.'

They remarked on how special their baby was to them:

> 'He was such a good baby – no trouble at all.'

And

> 'Everyone said how special she was.'

One relative referred to their 'little angel'.

All the mothers I spoke to described their babies in very positive terms. They spontaneously recalled many pleasant episodes of caring for their infants; this 'care' took many forms. They described the things they had provided for their children. Some described the efforts spent in preparing a nursery and getting ready for the arrival of the new infant. Some mentioned giving up work, or reducing their working hours in order to spend more time with their infants, thereby drawing attention to the way that motherhood had shaped and influenced other decisions. Others described specific activities associated with mothering that they had enjoyed. Some of these were essentially pleasurable activities, such as playing with, cuddling or talking to their infant. One mother spoke of her particular enjoyment at bathing her baby. For others, the activities they described might not be viewed by others as intrinsically enjoyable, but the association with their new identity as 'mothers' made them inherently part of the mothering experience, an experience that they themselves described as pleasurable. So, one mother described the enjoyment she derived from tidying up her infant's toys and clothes at the end of the day. She made the comment:

> 'I felt like a real mother when I was putting his things away at the end of the day – so ordinary and yet so special.'

Another mother described 'making up the feeds' as an enjoyable task. This example underlines the positive association mothers made between mundane tasks and caring for their infant. The daily tasks associated with looking after their babies were both enjoyable and meaningful for these mothers. In Western society, mothers not only care for their babies within the home, but they are also responsible for introducing their infants to the wider world.

Infants are part of families but not often viewed as part of a wide social circle. Mothers as carers are generally charged with representing their infant to others outside the immediate circle of family and friends. As part of this process, mothers often engage in mediating the impression their baby makes on others. Hence if a baby constantly cries whilst in company, the mother will often attempt to explain the cause of crying, such as 'he's tired' or 'she is not herself today'. Alternatively, they may place the crying in a wider context, such as 'she is not usually like this'. Mothers are constantly engaged in working to mediate the way that their children are presented to the world, contextualising their infant's behaviour and helping others to see their children in the best possible way, as well as seeking to minimise the disturbances their infants make, and attending to their needs.

This 'work' of representing their infants to others is an integral part of motherhood. It is part of the 'love story' that surrounds the loss of an infant with SIDS, in that mothers still seek to find ways to link their infant to the wider world. They may do this by engaging in activities to remember their infants, but also to remind others of the importance of the infant within the family and the subsequent loss that has been experienced. It has been suggested that in the West there is a hierarchy of loss in that the deaths of older children and young adults are often perceived as a greater or more significant loss than losses in old age or at the beginning of life.[10] Literature suggests that parents who lose a child at the beginning of life, through miscarriage, stillbirth or even infant death, are expected to come to terms with their loss more rapidly than the parents of older children; this is sometimes associated with a belief that a further pregnancy may mitigate the loss of an infant.[11] Therefore there are different social responses to the loss of an infant compared with the loss of an older child. This may be partly due to the extent to which an older child has social recognition outside the home and has developed relationships with people outside the family. However, the mothers I came into contact with throughout my study emphasised the huge void and sense of loss brought about by the death of a young child.

Sudden loss

SIDS stands for 'sudden infant death syndrome'. The suddenness of the death is highly significant. Babies who die of SIDS are generally not unwell, although sometimes retrospectively there may have been significant changes in health.[12] The suddenness of the death is particularly difficult to cope with. Some mothers commented that they worried that they had missed something significant – one said:

> 'I went over that last day in my head, again and again, looking for some clue as to what was going to happen.'

This is a remark which resonates with comments made by Sarah Murphy in her book *Coping with Cot Death* written after her own daughter died of SIDS.[13] She wrote a poem about her grief, a year after her baby died, reflecting on the suddenness of the death and the awfulness of her loss. She re-visits the day her baby died and considers whether she missed any changes in her child. She comments on how mothers may scrutinise their own actions for something they may have missed, searching for a reason for the death. She conveys very well the shock of a sudden, unexpected death, with no apparent prior indication of what was to come. She states:

> 'In our rational minds we know that there is nothing we could have done to prevent the death, and that we are not to blame in any way, but in our hearts we feel we must be to blame because healthy, well-protected babies don't die suddenly for no reason.'

Other parents have also written poems and reflections about their babies and the shock of the suddenness of the death is often mentioned. These reflections on their experiences of SIDS are frequently shared by mothers via self-help websites and self-help groups established for those whose infants have died.[14] Some of these reflect on whether if they had known that they would have so little time together, or even known that it was their last day together, they would have done anything differently. Murphy concludes that she regrets deeply:

'. . . the photographs I never took, the moments I never captured, those many other moments that I wasted on household chores and trivia, and which I could have spent with Elizabeth if only I had known how little time we would have together.'

However, mothers also reflect on the positive memories too. One of the mothers I interviewed stated:

'I feel desperate at what has happened – I loved her so much – and even the day she died, we had had a lovely morning together – I hold onto that in my mind.'

Murphy comments:

'. . . when the baby has very little past, that past becomes very precious indeed.'

Mothers were often the ones who first discovered that their baby had died. For some this discovery was made when they went to wake them in the morning. One mother recounted feeling pleased that her infant had 'slept through' and not woken in the night only to find that her baby had died. Another mother described going to wake her son from an afternoon nap and the 'sickening' discovery that he could not be roused. One mother I spoke to described how she returned from making a phone call to find her infant had died on the sofa. These descriptions conveyed quite graphically the unexpected suddenness of the death, and the rapid transition from a normal to traumatic day. The feelings of responsibility for the care of the infant, which accompany motherhood, caused these mothers to revisit those last moments repeatedly and sometimes to question their own mothering. This occurred in spite of the fact that the death was subsequently categorised as SIDS, which meant that the children had not died of an identifiable cause. Sarah Murphy reflected in particular on the sense of responsibility she felt, because her daughter had died whilst in her care.

'This can't be happening . . .'

Many mothers described the sequence of events from the point at which they found that their baby had died. Some described finding their baby dead and knowing straight away that the baby had died. They described attempting resuscitation themselves, or watching a relative try to resuscitate the baby, and calling the emergency services who then took over the resuscitation attempt. One mother described her efforts as:

> '. . . doing everything I could, for as long as I could, and knowing that it wouldn't do any good, but needing to do something.'

Some mothers outlined the mixed emotions they felt in allowing themselves to hope that their first impressions were wrong and that the baby could be successfully resuscitated only to later have their worst fears confirmed. One mother described the experience as a 'rollercoaster', whilst another said it felt as:

> '. . . though time had stopped and was totally suspended yet really long at the same time.'

Some mothers described the agonising wait for the ambulance to arrive whilst they continued their desperate efforts to resuscitate their infant. Some of the mothers described the journey to the hospital and in particular the long wait for news, sitting outside the resuscitation room.

The descriptions of the space in which they waited, and the length of time which they had to wait, featured strongly in their stories of helplessness, and captured their feelings of being in a state of limbo waiting for news. One mother commented on how she felt: 'suspended from time' and surrounded by: 'very busy people, but with nothing at all for me to do'. This feeling of powerlessness and disembodiment from what was going on around her seemed to capture the essence of the waiting period. Some writers[15] have commented on how the attempts at resuscitation following SIDS are helpful to parents, as it gives them time to adjust to the loss of their infant. However, the women I interviewed who mentioned that period of time, described it as a time of confusion. Many of the mothers described the feelings of vulnerability that they experienced at the hospital, and the awfulness of 'not knowing'. They outlined the huge contrast between the busyness of the hospital staff involved in the resuscitation attempt, and the isolation and inactivity of those who have to sit and wait. Stefan Timmermans refers to the protocols that emergency staff are expected to follow in relation to SIDS cases, describing how all sudden infant deaths are subject to a resuscitation attempt.[16] This might prove helpful to parents later as they are assured that 'everything was done that could be done', but my conversations with mothers indicated that this activity also gives the parents a false sense of hope at the time, destabilising the conclusions that they had already reached, and encouraging them to 'hope beyond hope' that their first impressions were wrong, only to have these hopes dashed.

In recent years much work has been done on trying to find ways to ease the transition for families at the impending loss of a loved one. Relatives are often called into hospital to be present at the end of life and to offer support to their loved one and often to each other. It is thought that involvement in care can help with accepting the reality of the death and with the mourning process.

In cases of SIDS, often the opposite happens, the baby is taken from the parents for resuscitation and they are excluded from the proceedings. At a time when they could be spending time with, and taking their leave of, their infant, they are instead waiting in a hospital corridor for news. The mother may be unaware of what the process of resuscitation may entail. One mother, speaking at a conference I attended, graphically described calling the ambulance to a baby who was dead but had the appearance of being peacefully asleep, and contrasting this with being called back in to see her baby in hospital and being aware of the 'bruising and discolouration' of his body, which she attributed to the resuscitation process.

Some mothers described the time spent in the hospital with their infants after the resuscitation attempt. One described sitting with her husband just holding the baby and not wanting to go home. Most of the mothers I met described not wanting to leave their baby. The mothers I talked to also described their distress at leaving their babies alone; some also mentioned the 'coldness' of the chapel of rest. These comments relate to the physical aspects of the mothering relationship: one of the accepted roles of a mother is to ensure that their babies are always warm and well cared for, and the stark contrast between this and having to leave their babies alone in a cold chapel of rest was palpable. Pamela Elder writing about the loss of her teenage daughter commented on the difficulty of leaving her daughter for the last time, but also of noting how she looked as though she was asleep. This increased her difficulty in assimilating that her daughter had died.[3] Some mothers who talked to me about their experiences also commented on how their babies looked as if they were 'just asleep' or 'about to wake up any minute'. They too recounted how this added to the difficulty of leaving them. The appearance of the baby as 'asleep' is reinforced by photographs taken after the death of babies who have died.

One mother showed me a photograph of her infant taken in the chapel of rest and described the situation in which the photograph of her baby was taken. She commented that she wished that she had taken more pictures when the baby was alive, saying:

'We didn't because I suppose we were busy with living then.'

Another mother showed me a photograph of a family group with the baby at the centre, explaining that the photograph was taken after the death. These pictures demonstrated their continued maternal relationship, as the photograph was very similar to the photographs often taken at christenings and other family events.[17]

Being with the baby

One of the ways in which mothers expressed their love for their infants was through recalling the places and times that emphasised their sense of loss. The mothers I interviewed described different locations that they associated with expressions of their maternal love and the overwhelming desire to be with their infants. Mothers also described the way in which they engaged in activities at different sites that helped them to express their love for their infants. One of these sites was the chapel of rest. One mother described visiting her daughter at the chapel of rest to sit with her, and taking a gift with her to place in her little daughter's coffin. This mother was disturbed to find the post mortem scars when she touched her daughter. These scars were a tangible reminder of the indignities to which the tiny body had been subjected, and a clear indication of the way in which other people had handled her baby.[18]

As I talked to mothers whose infants had died I was aware of the many references they made to touch, smell and sometimes even taste, indicating their heightened senses at the time. Mothers commented on the scents they associated with their infant's death, and some of these were more positive than others. One woman described the all-pervasive smell of lavender when she visited the chapel of rest and said:

'That smell will always remind me of that time, just sitting there with the smell of lavender on the breeze.'

For another, the smell of hospital disinfectant led her to recall her time waiting in casualty:

> 'I think that smell will always take me back to the uncertainty and hope of those moments.'

The association of events and scents seemed to typify the responsibilities of motherhood and the love of these mothers for their babies. It is another example of how the extraordinariness of a sudden unanticipated death becomes attached to very ordinary scents – and from that point on renders them highly significant. Likewise mothers commented on the texture of objects around them. One commented on 'the cold touch of the bricks' in the chapel of rest. Another mentioned 'the stiffness of the hospital sheet' when she went to see her baby in a room at Accident & Emergency. Others referred to the sensory experiences of touching their babies: 'stroking her hair – always so soft', or 'holding his little hand and foot'. The links between senses and experiences potentially become triggers to recalling the specificities of those events.

The funeral

The mothers I met expressed their love for their infant in many different ways. They often described the funeral of their baby as important, not just as a part of the grieving process, but also as an expression of love. They outlined many different aspects of the funeral and its importance to them as mothers, including aspects such as the flowers, the location, the music and the service itself. The importance of the funeral included the opportunity for recognition of the infant outside the immediate family, as well as being an occasion for them to represent their infant to others and demonstrate their baby's importance within the family. Funerals also provided a particular space for them to remember specific aspects of the baby's life and to support one another. It seemed that it was very important to mothers that other people acknowledged their infants.

Some mothers commented on the number of people who attended the funeral. This was described in terms of the extent to which other people were affected by the child's life and death. This recognition of the child outside the immediate family may be important in that the infant is generally known only within the context of the family, and the presence of non-family members at the funeral places the baby within a wider social context, and acknowledges their life as a part of society. This acknowledgement took different forms. One woman commented:

'A lot of friends came – there were lots of people there.'

Some women commented on particular people who attended, and the attendance of people outside of the family was particularly important. For example, one mother mentioned the importance for her of healthcare staff attending the funeral, and another commented on the fact that her health visitor was there. Mothers acknowledged that other people would find the funeral of a baby difficult, but appreciated the support of people they knew.

For some mothers the floral tributes were comforting, not only for their appearance, but also as an expression of love, acknowledgement and support. One mother commented on the floral tributes at the funeral:

'There were flowers everywhere, a blur of colour – they smelled wonderful too . . . comforting and sad at the same time.'

Another commented:

'I think I will always be able to close my eyes and smell that lovely smell, there were so many flowers that the perfume filled the whole place.'

Another relative felt that:

'All those vibrant colours seemed to remind us that this was a young and active little person, full of life.'

The image and scent of the flowers was a significant element of their story about SIDS – the flowers representative of something much deeper and meaningful. Condolence cards were sometimes also mentioned – mothers seemed to find letters of condolence and cards helpful in making visible the relationships they and their baby had with others around them.

Many mothers conveyed how difficult they found the day of the funeral. One mother described how numb she felt at the funeral:

'I could hear voices, but they seemed distant almost like the voices you hear at a swimming pool, it was like I was there but also somewhere else.'

This strange sense of disembodiment and unreality was shared by other women – who described a variety of feelings of 'separateness' and also described feeling bereft, isolated and remote from what was going on around them. One mother commented that it was like watching herself in a play saying:

'It didn't feel real . . . it was only later that reality set in.'

Another mother commented:

'I felt like only a part of me was actually there – another part of me was hovering somewhere above (the proceedings) just watching it all.'

A mother whose baby had died some years previously commented:

'You need to feel the pain, tablets and medicines – even drink . . . can make you detached for a while, but it doesn't make the pain go away; hard as the funeral is, it is important to feel it all.'

Sometimes mothers commented on the funeral itself and how the various elements of the funeral were ways of expressing their love for their baby as well as saying goodbye. This expression included choosing the clothes the baby was to be buried in, jewellery and toys which were placed with the baby, and features of the service itself, such as flowers and music. More than one mother described the plans for the funeral as being an opportunity to demonstrate their love for their infant – making remarks such as:

'There was no expense spared'
and
'We did everything as nicely as we could.'

A place to love . . .

Many things were said that interested me during the interviews, including the comments mothers made about reminiscence and the intentional remembering of their babies. They talked about choosing times and places to particularly remember their baby. For some this was part of a routine involving an activity associated with remembering, whereas for others the opportunity to remember was associated with particular triggers that were used in both planned and spontaneous ways. A pattern seemed to emerge from their comments that identified three main areas that were particularly important sites for remembering the infants: the home, objects relating to the baby, and visits to the grave.

Remembering at home

Many authors have described how, when a person dies, the family leave the room or the possessions of the deceased just where they have been left or placed by that person.[19] However, the situation may be very different when a baby dies. Babies' bedrooms or nurseries have generally been put together by parents, often in anticipation of the arrival of a child. Unlike older children and adults, the baby has not determined the layout of their room or the placement of objects in that space. So it would seem that for some parents the need to preserve the room as it was is less important and the individual objects are more important than the room. Babies' possessions also have a way of infiltrating the whole household, so the evidence of their presence within the family may be everywhere. Sometimes the baby shares the parents' bedroom in the early months of life; sometimes they share a room with an older sibling. In these situations it may not be practical to leave the baby's room untouched. It would seem from my conversations with mothers that it is relatively unusual to preserve a room intact following SIDS, but that is not to say that parents do not preserve the imprint of their infants on the home and the family. There is another issue to consider here too: although the infant bedroom may be associated with many happy times and memories of mothering, it may also be associated with finding the baby dead.

Occasionally mothers described these powerful images of their dead infant. One commented:

> 'Sometimes when I close my eyes I can see him lying there with his face discoloured and pale . . . it's not how I want to remember, but it is often the image that comes to me first.'

These images were described as difficult to eradicate. Some of the mothers I interviewed told me how they had wanted to get rid of the cot soon after the death. One mother said:

> 'Every time I saw it, I could see (her) lying there and felt a sense of despair and helplessness all over again.'[20]

Another mother felt she had to change the space 'for the sake of my other children'. Some authors have written about the way in which mothers whose children die often dispose of objects quite soon after the death.[21] However, I found that this was not the case with the mothers I talked to; although they may have changed the bedroom, they had kept a range of objects relating to their babies.

One even mentioned the difficulty of throwing anything away at all:

> 'I found it hard to throw away half-used packets of baby food or baby bath, there was just something awful in parting with any of it, it was a link to her, and I didn't want to lose any of those links.'

Other mothers described how they were continually finding objects that reminded them of their infants. I came to think of this as being 'ambushed' by grief – the unplanned exposure to triggers that caused them to focus their thoughts on their infants. This was different to the way in which they kept objects that were collected together and used to actively remember their infants.[22]

There has been a lot written about the importance of objects and their place in engendering emotions. Deborah Lupton (1998)[23] describes how objects can be used to define a 'territory of the self', in which material objects indicate aspects of the self which one wishes to convey to others. One of the powerful examples she uses is the way that, in everyday life, mothers take photographs of their children and objects made by their children to work – thereby making their motherhood visible in a child-free space. Other writers, such as Daniel Miller (1987)[24], suggest that individuals often surround themselves with objects that are 'inspirational', or indicative of a lifestyle or attributes that they would like to acquire. In similar ways, the objects bought for babies may also contribute to maternal identity or reflect the parental aspirations for their child. There are many references in literature to the importance of 'love tokens' or 'love gifts' – items that remind the recipient of the object of their affections. These objects could be described as linking the two parties together, and reminders of an affectional bond. Inese Wheeler (1998)[25] researched the importance of 'link objects' in the grief of those who had lost a child. Link objects were described as objects that parents used to actively remember their child, such as photographs, toys, clothes and other possessions. She reported how parents responded to and used these objects, including stroking, holding and kissing objects.

The importance of objects became increasingly apparent to me throughout the research interviews. The women I interviewed described how they had collected objects together that reminded them of their infants and their mothering. They described the purposeful putting together of a range of objects in one place, sometimes a toy box, sometimes a drawer or other receptacle.

Sometimes these objects were chosen for their appearance. Photographs were frequently used as link objects. Photographs are able to evoke a memory extremely powerfully, and as such are highly significant in grief,[26] some of which I will touch on later. The photographs mothers showed me often included an image of their infant with a loved toy. The mothers sometimes showed me the toys that featured in the photographs. The sight and texture of a teddy bear or other soft toy evoked strong memories of their infants, and the objects were handled with great care. Other objects that seemed important because of their appearance included clothing and sometimes jewellery purchased for the infant. The mothers I met sometimes told me about the origins of the object in question, when or where it was bought, or who gave it to the infant. I felt that in doing this they were affirming a sense of importance and place to their infants by recalling loving relationships between their infant and others. These were items that had been carefully chosen and selected by themselves or others for their infant, or objects associated with pleasant memories.

As well as looking at and sometimes handling objects, some mothers also smelled the objects relating to their babies. On one occasion the mother I was talking to reached into a box and drew out a bag containing the baby's bed sheets. The bag was carefully knotted, but she untied it and smelled the contents, before handing the bag to me. The implication was clear, I too was being invited to smell the contents. As I took hold of that plastic bag, a whole range of emotions overtook me – this mother was prepared to share something really significant and personal with me. The smell of those bedclothes at once transported me back to my own mothering experiences. It was the smell of bath time and bedtime – a unique nursery scent, lending something to the combined perfumes of infant, baby bath and baby powder.[27] In smelling those bedclothes I was thinking not about her baby, so much as about my own – and in that moment I had a particular resonance with her: two mothers sitting together on a wintry afternoon, being reminded evocatively of what it feels like to be a mother. It was a unique and unifying moment – a moment of solidarity, which immediately dissolved into a new insight into something of the enormity of her loss. It was an action that conveyed so much, and all without words. Words were not even necessary. Some stories are visual. This particular love story certainly was.

As mothers showed me their objects and talked about their importance, their hands and body movements told a particular story of love and loss. As mothers showed me these objects, they occasionally cuddled or held particular toys against their cheek, or cradled them in their arms. Some kissed photographs they had shown me before putting them back into their place. Toys were often patted, cuddled and caressed, photographs stroked, clothes shaken out and carefully refolded with great care. Jewellery was held and admired, and everyday objects such as cups and cutlery held, and the weight felt in the hands before being gently replaced. I was acutely aware of the tactile parts of remembering, the stroking, rocking, caressing, which in itself reminded me of activities associated with mothering as they mirrored the actions of maternal care.

One of the ways in which mothers tell stories of their experiences of SIDS is to talk about the positive experiences of mothering their children. Self-help-group websites for parents whose children have died of SIDS are filled with reminiscences and shared memories of happy times shared with their infants. Because children who die of SIDS are by definition two years of age or younger, these shared memories often focus around the day-to-day relationship between mother and infant, rather than a host of special events. The time factor generally mitigates against many shared celebrations, holidays, festivals and other events. Hence many of the poems and 'in memoriam' comments posted on websites dwell on the enjoyment derived from the infant's company, and the pleasures of play and care that intersperse the routine care of the infant. This is one of the key elements of the love story that mothers tell about their relationship with their infants. They describe the pleasure and enjoyment derived from the 'ordinariness' of their activities. This ranged from just enjoying being with the baby and engaging in everyday activities, to the pleasure derived in being identified as a 'mother'. One of the participants at a bereavement group put this into words:

> 'I waited a long time to be a mother, and I just enjoyed being a mum . . . and being able to tell other people that I was a mum.'

For some women, motherhood is a longed-for identity – which is suddenly disrupted by the death of their infant. Another mother referred to this loss of identity as a mother, when her baby died. She described the importance to her of going to the local park to feed the ducks and continuing an activity that had been part of her identity as a mother, she commented:

> 'I still go there, because I have been a mother and I will be again.'

Mothers and mothering

The theme of still being a 'mother', but not having a child to mother, was a recurrent one, particularly for those women who had lost their only child. However, it was also important for mothers who had other children, in that they articulated that it was important to be seen as a mother to the child who had died. One mother summed this up by saying:

> 'People say when they are introducing me to friends, this is Carol with her two (children) and I want to say "I have three children, I am a mother of three, but one has died."'

This statement encapsulates an important part of maternal identity – in that mothers need others to acknowledge their mothering relationship with each child. Mothering and the identity of mother is regarded and formed in relation to each of their offspring and not as a single identity. Therefore it is important to note that women cannot be simply categorised as 'mothers' or 'no-longer mothers' because the situation is more complex and messy than those simple categorisations allow. The lack of ongoing recognition of these women as mothers is highly problematic for the women concerned, and leads them to engage in particular work to demonstrate and reaffirm their identity as mothers. This is the challenge for women whose only children die of SIDS, in finding ways to continue and maintain their identity as a mother in the absence of an infant or child. In her work on miscarriage and stillbirth, Alice Lovell comments that a death at the beginning of life can sometimes be viewed by society as 'cancelling out' the birth.[28] Mothers engage in particular work to ensure that their infant is remembered and valued, and that their identity as mother to their baby is maintained.

I am not claiming here that all mothers feel the same way about their identity following the loss of a child, but rather to look for patterns and similarities in what mothers have said about their grief experience following SIDS, whilst at the same time acknowledging the differences that will also exist.

A space for expression

Many of the mothers I spoke to described a need to talk about and express their identity as mothers and their love for their infants. The places for such expression were varied. Some of the women I met found self-help groups and the company of other women whose children had died a positive environment in which to talk about their infants. Many organisations have been established to provide this type of space to talk about loss of a child.[29] One of the repeated patterns that emerged in my conversations with women whose infants had died, and with some of the professionals who worked with these women, was the difficulty encountered in talking about their experiences to other people. There is a general reluctance within the population to engage in conversation with those who have experienced bereavement, particularly the sudden loss of a child. Part of this may be due to an anxiety about 'saying the wrong thing' or feeling inadequate in saying anything. But some mothers also felt that they had come to represent 'the worst thing that can happen', i.e. losing a child, and as such were a constant reminder to other mothers of the fragility of life. Some mothers felt that the commonality they shared with other women in some of their social groups was that they had children of similar ages, and suddenly with the death of their baby there was a perception that the commonality had gone. This is perhaps even more acute in that many women on leaving work to have a baby make friends with other women in similar situations via parentcraft classes and clinic attendances, and later through mother and toddler groups. Assumptions were also sometimes made that bereaved mothers would not want to be with other mothers and infants following the death of their own child.[30] It would seem that just when women need the most support, people feel the least able to give it.

The women I met overcame these obstacles to talking about their infant in various ways. They identified particular places where they could reminisce about their infant, either on their own or in the company of others. Some became involved in self-help groups, either by personal attendance or as part of a virtual community (such as posting a memorial notice on a website), as well as reminiscing on their own. Some mentioned talking to strangers about the loss of their infant – and finding this was helpful. This was often in response to someone initiating a conversation as to how they were feeling. For other mothers the urge to talk about their infant and their loss suddenly overcame them. The following comment was made by a woman I met who had lost an infant, but was also explaining her role as a representative of a support group aimed at helping other women whose infants had died:

> 'I was in a shop, buying some socks of all things . . . suddenly I felt overwhelmed with the need to tell the shop assistant about what had happened to me . . . I passed the socks to her, but didn't let go, there we were both holding onto these socks and I was telling her about what happened to me. She just seemed so sympathetic, something about her . . . it sounds really odd, but it was okay.'

Another woman described telling someone at a bus stop about what had happened:

'It just suddenly tumbled out – once I started to talk I couldn't stop . . .'

The unburdening of themselves to strangers seemed to be quite cathartic and appeared to help them overcome the difficulty of being able to talk to others about their loss. Some of the mothers I interviewed commented that they had found it helpful to have the opportunity to talk to me about their baby and what had happened to them.

'I go to the grave to be with him'

Some mothers also felt that the specific place of burial was really important. One mother described how she had chosen a grave which was near to her grandmother:

'I feel as though she will be looking after her.'

This was an important sentiment for her, and familiar or pleasant locations were mentioned as important by other mothers. This is a seeming continuation of maternal care, placing the baby in a 'good' place or close to the grave of a relative. It conveyed a sense of continued care, but also of choosing a significant place. One woman described how she pictured her child 'asleep on the hillside' going on to say 'it is a nice place'.

In my conversations with these mothers, a number of references to the infant graves and their different relationships to the graves emerged. For some of the mothers the grave was described in terms of being an extension of the household. For example, one mother commented about the frequency of her visits to the grave, stating:

'I clean the house, and then we come here and I tidy the grave. I sort out the flowers and tidy things up and then just stay for a while.'

For this mother, the physical care of the grave was an expression of care. In the same way that she described caring for her home, and thereby caring for her family, she described caring for the grave and so continued to 'care for' her infant. She went on to say that her mother also visited the grave frequently:

'She sometimes gets there before me and starts tidying it up, moving the leaves and so on . . . I don't really like her doing it . . . I try to get there first . . . it's my job you see, I'm the mum.'

For this mother the grave was a site for expression of love and care via physical activities. She also described spending time just being at the grave once the 'housekeeping' type of activities were completed. This gives some insight into some of the ways the grave becomes a site for different types of expression of love and care. Sometimes taking flowers and occasionally toys to the grave was mentioned as important. More than one mother mentioned talking to the baby whilst at the grave, and another of the women I talked to described singing or humming to her baby whilst at the grave.

On one occasion I spoke to a friend of the bereaved family. She talked about the grave of her friend's baby. She described it as containing flowers, toys and 'windmills', the small wind-driven toys on sticks so beloved of many small children. She described the grave as:

'Very much the grave of a child, bright and cheerful'
adding
'. . . if a grave can be considered cheerful.'

It seemed to me that the mother had created a child-friendly space, even in a graveyard.[31] The toys and flowers were an expression of her love for her baby, and also contributed to her ongoing identity as a mother.

The notion of 'child-friendly' spaces for expression also seemed significant in my conversations with mothers. One of the mothers described taking her other children to the grave, and how they rearranged and played with the toys whilst they were there. This seemed a significant part of viewing the infant as an ongoing part of the family, and for this mother it was important to encourage her other children to be involved in activities. Their participation in tidying the grave also helped to associate the visits with an enjoyable activity and even associate the grave with play. Cemeteries and graveyards in contemporary society are not generally associated with actions other than relatively formal activities to do with remembering the deceased or caring for the plot. But this description of play and child activity – along with the descriptions of some of the graves as child-friendly places – seemed to resonate with some historical accounts of cemeteries in which graves were more closely associated with the activities of everyday life, and there was less of a division between the worlds of the living and the dead.[32,33]

One mother summed up her visits to the grave by stating:

> 'I go to the grave to be with him.'

This is not a sentiment which is particular to SIDS; there are other accounts of this sense of 'visiting' the deceased.[34] But it is a sentiment that expresses some of the importance of having a place to express love to the lost family member through activities, gifts or conversation, whether this is at a grave, or some other significant place chosen as a site for memorial or reminiscence.

Reminiscence

In addition to the graves there were other places that mothers described as significant in reminiscing and remembering their

infant. As already mentioned, some mothers described how particular activities such as visits to the park were times for reflection.
Returning to places they had visited with the baby was a focus for
remembering and reminiscence. Likewise, mothers reported that
negative memories had become associated with other venues; one
commented that the hospital was now associated for her with the
final confirmation that her baby had died:

> 'I find it difficult to get it out of my mind when I go anywhere
> near there.'

For another, she felt she couldn't easily enter the room in the
house where the baby had died without 'seeing', for a moment, the
incident all over again.

So, the women I met could clearly differentiate between the
reminiscence that they set out to embark upon, in that they were
choosing to remember their infant by using particular triggers –
objects or visits to places, and the incidences that triggered grief in
an unplanned way. Sometimes reminiscence was described as
being focused around particular triggers such as possessions
belonging to the baby or objects associated with the infant
(which I will discuss in a later chapter). These triggers could be
used by mothers to facilitate episodes of remembering at times and
places that they felt were private and therefore appropriate.
Mothers also mentioned using photographs to remember their
infant.[35]

By contrast, some mothers described the way that they were
sometimes surprised by grief, in that a sudden reminiscence caught
them unawares and could be difficult to manage. Examples of this
included being reminded of a particular incident or coming across
an object which belonged to their infant. Anne Diamond, in her
account of the loss of her son Sebastian, describes coming across
one of his socks in the pocket of a dress she had not worn for some
time and being suddenly overwhelmed by grief.[36] The mothers I
talked to seemed to find these grief reactions particularly difficult if
they felt that they were in a place where they were unable to
express their distress and sorrow in private, or where others would

not understand their reaction. One of the mothers I met described moving a sofa and finding a baby's sock underneath and feeling overcome with emotion. Another mentioned constantly coming across items connected with her baby in the days after the death, from packets of baby food in the kitchen cupboard to the baby bubble-bath in the bathroom. The capacity of these very ordinary objects to underline the enormity of loss is indicative of the depth of grief that these women had to cope with.

Using their name

Many of the mothers I interviewed also mentioned the importance of being able to say the baby's name in conversation. As already mentioned, social conventions and anxieties surrounding the way people interact with the bereaved in the Western world leads to people avoiding the mention of the baby's name or reference to the baby for fear of upsetting the bereaved mother. Hilka Laakso and Pauhonen-Ilomen (2001) describe how this sometimes may extend into ridding the home of items that might trigger grief, or putting them out of sight.[21, 37] Some of the women I talked to commented on how much they wanted to talk about their baby or hear the baby's name mentioned. One commented that:

> 'The befriender[38] always uses his name – it's something they do, they always use their name.'

Another mother commented:

> 'I like it when I hear people use their name.'

These mothers indicated that they regarded using the baby's name as part of good practice, but also that doing so represented an acknowledgement of their infant and their own sense of loss and a personalisation of care.

Representing motherhood

One of the ways in which some mothers expressed their ongoing love for their infants was in attempting to maintain some of the physical effects of motherhood. This seemed to be associated with issues of identity as mothers, but also in fostering an ongoing connection to their infant. One woman described how she had been breastfeeding her infant, and following the death had been offered medication, and advised to cut back on her fluids to reduce the production of breast milk. She described how she had resisted doing this as she felt that continued lactation, even if for only a short time, was a link with the baby. Hence she was prepared to cope with the discomfort of lactation, rather than intervene to interrupt her supply of milk. One could argue that her actions meant that she was continuing to be a mothering body – a body which physically had adapted to the needs of the infant.

Another mother described how she had put weight on in pregnancy and was keen to lose the additional weight up until the point at which her baby died. She then described how the weight was associated with pregnancy and motherhood and 'didn't seem so bad'. Thus her weight problem became primarily seen as a side-effect of her mothering rather than in the more negative ways weight gain is often perceived. It has to be emphasised that these women were quite recently bereaved, and may have felt differently over time. The emphasis on bodies as 'mothering bodies' interprets (uncomfortable and possibly unwanted) bodily changes into a necessary part of the mothering process, a biological process with which mothers readily comply and accommodate for the sake of the baby. Hence, reproduction itself and its physical effects and consequences are re-configured as an act of motherly love.

The love story told by mothers whose infants have died of SIDS is varied and complex, multiple rather than singular. But it is a story of a deep love for their children that is made visible in many ways, some to do with the context and places, but also relating to their bodies. It is a story of love for an infant that impacts all areas of the mother's life – identity, actions, emotions and the physical body – and it is the loss of this loving relationship that in turn affects all of those areas. Whilst there may be a focus by many on the emotional effects of loss, this does not minimise the other significant and sudden changes brought about by the loss of the child. Women do offer to tell their stories of these changes, but they may not always be heard. It is a challenge to think about the potential gap between the stories people tell of their grief and the stories we really listen to and so actually hear. There are stories that are epic in scale, such as the love story of maternal grief, and they are so often publicly condensed into short stories, simply because society doesn't take time to hear them. The reluctance to really listen to those who grieve may mean that these stories become 'backstage' rather than widely shared.[39]

Notes and references

1 Hallam E, Hockey J, Howarth G, editors. *Beyond the Body: death and social identity*. London: Routledge; 1999.

2 Littlewood J. Just an old fashioned love song or a 'harlequin romance'? Some experiences of widowhood. In: Hockey J, Katz J, Small N, editors. *Grief, Mourning and Death Ritual*. Buckingham: Open University Press; 2001.

3 Elder PA. Portrait of family grief. In: Weston R, Martin P, Anderson Y, editors. *Loss and Bereavement: managing change*. London: Blackwell Scientific; 1998.

4 For example, Gloria Hunniford, writing about the death of her daughter Caron Keating, also describes her special relationship with her daughter from birth to death and beyond as an enduring love:
Hunniford G. *Next to you: Caron's courage remembered by her mother*. London: Penguin; 2005.
See also relevant bereavement texts:
Archer J. *The Nature of Grief: the evolution and psychology of reactions to loss*. London: Routledge; 1999.
Cleiren M, PhD. *Bereavement and Adaptation: a comparative study of the aftermath of death*. Washington, USA: Hemisphere Press; 1993.
Cline S. *Lifting the Taboo: women, death and dying*. London: Little & Brown; 1995.
Corr C, Corr D. *Handbook of Childhood Death and Bereavement*. New York: Springer; 1996.
Currer C. *Responding to Grief: dying, bereavement and social care*. London: Palgrave; 2001.

5 'Other' meaning different to general social norms.

6 See Chapter 1 for the Beckwith definition of SIDS; there are also other

definitions, including World Health Organization and ICD classifications.

7 Murphy and others refer specifically to the 'suddenness' of death.

8 In many contexts it is now viewed as good nursing practice to encourage family members to remain with dying relatives, including, at times, during resuscitation.

See also:

Oliviere D, Hargreaves R, Monroe B. *Good Practices in Palliative Care*. Aldershot: Ashgate; 1998.

Timmermans S. Resuscitation technology in the emergency department: towards a dignified death. *Sociol Health Illn*. 1998; **20**(2): 144–67.

9 See Bowlby's work on attachment:

Bowlby J. *Loss, Sadness and Depression*. London: Penguin; 1968.

Bowlby J. *The Making and Breaking of Affectional Bonds*. London: Tavistock; 1979.

10 See Hallam, Hockey & Howarth for a discussion on the boundaries between physical death and social death, and Lovell for comment on the social experience of death at the beginning of life:

Hallam E, Hockey J, Howarth G, editors. *Beyond the Body: death and social identity*. London: Routledge; 1999.

Lovell A. Death at the beginning of life. In: Field D, Hockey J and Small N, editors. *Death, Gender and Ethnicity*. London: Routledge; 2001.

11 Small N, Hockey J. Discourse into practice: the production of bereavement care. In: Hockey J, Katz J, Small N, editors. *Grief, mourning and death ritual*. Buckingham: Open University Press; 1997.

For perspectives on parental experiences of grief see:

Cline S. *Lifting the Taboo: women, death and dying*. London: Little & Brown; 1995.

Dent A, Condon L, Blair P *et al*. A study of bereavement after a sudden and unexpected infant death. *Arch Dis Child*. 1996; **74**(6): 522–6.

Mirren E, editor. *Our Children: coming to terms with the loss of a child*. London: Hodder & Stoughton; 1984.

Stewart A, Dent A. *At a Loss: bereavement care when a baby dies*. London: Balliere Tindall; 1994.

12 For exploration of retrospective identification of risk factors/indicators associated with SIDS see:

Blair PS, Fleming PJ, Leach CEA *et al*. A clinical comparison of SIDS and explained sudden infant deaths: how healthy and how normal. *Arch Dis Child*. 2000; **82**(2): 98–106.

Blair PS, Nadin P, Fleming PJ *et al*. Weight gain and sudden infant death syndrome: changes in weight z scores may identify infants at increased risk. *Arch Dis Child*. 2000; **82**(6): 462–9.

For work on risk factors associated with SIDS see also:

Cole TJ, Gilbert RE, Fleming PJ *et al*. Baby Check and the Avon Infant Mortality Study. *Arch Dis Child*. 1991; **66**(9): 1077–8.

De Jonge GA, Engelberts AC, Koomen-Liefting AJ. Cot death and prone sleeping position in The Netherlands. *BMJ*. 1989; **298**(6675): 722.

Dwyer T, Ponsonby AL, Newman NM *et al*. Prospective cohort study of prone sleeping position and sudden infant death syndrome. *Lancet*. 1991; **337**(8752): 12244–7.

Emery JL. Cot death on different days of the week. *Arch Dis Child*. 1998; **79**(2): 198.

Fleming PJ, Blair PS, Bacon C *et al*. Environment of infants during sleep and risk of sudden infant death syndrome: results of 1993–5 case control study for confidential enquiry into stillbirths and sudden deaths in infancy. *BMJ*. 1996; **313**(7051): 191–8.

Fleming PJ, Blair PS, Pollard K *et al*. Pacifier use and sudden infant death syndrome: results from the CSDI/SUDI case control study. *Arch Dis Child*. 1999; **81**(2): 112–6.

Fleming P, Blair P, Bacon C *et al*., editors. *Sudden Unexpected Deaths in Infancy: the CESDI SUDI studies 1993–1996*. London: The Stationery Office; 2000.

North K, Fleming P, Golding J. Pacifier use and morbidity in the first six months of life. *PMID*. 1999; **103**(3): E34.

13 Murphy S. *Coping with Cot Death*. London: Sheldon Press; 1990.

14 For examples see the FSID website: www.sids.org.uk/fsid/ (accessed 18 September 2006).

15 Timmermans S. Resuscitation technology in the emergency department: towards a dignified death. *Sociol Health Illn*. 1998; **20**(2): 144–67.

16 Participants in Timmermans' research stated that this protocol applied in the context of their work, even when they were certain that the infant was dead and beyond resuscitation.

17 Also discussed in a later chapter.

18 There was also a clear contrast between the mother's care of her baby and the interventions that followed, reinforcing the way in which the priorities of the medical services are emphasised over those of the parents.

19 For examples see:

Parkes CM. *Bereavement: studies of grief in adult life*. 2nd ed. Harmondsworth: Penguin; 1986.

Parkes CM. *Bereavement*. London: Tavistock; 1996.

Parkes CM. Introduction. In: Parkes CM, Markus A, editors. *Coping with Loss*. London: BMJ Books; 1998.

20 Some mothers spoke of wanting to destroy the cot, as they never wanted a baby to sleep in it again.

21 Laakso H, Pauhonen-Ilomen M. Mothers' experience of social support following the death of a child. *J Clin Nurs*. 2001; **2**: 176–86.
Murphy S. *Coping with Cot Death*. London: Sheldon Press; 1990.

22 There are similarities between the keeping of love letters from a romantic partner and the keeping of baby books by mothers, as both may be used to trigger positive emotions regarding the relationship and reminiscence/visualisation of the person.

23 Deborah Lupton's book is primarily a sociological book on the role of emotions in social life – and although it does not focus specifically on grief and grief experience, there are areas of her work which seem pertinent and relevant here. Lupton D, editor. *The Emotional Self: a sociocultural exploration*. London: Sage; 1998.

24 Miller D. *Material Culture and Mass Consumption*. Oxford: Blackwell; 1987.

25 Wheeler I. The role of linking objects in parental bereavement. *Omega (Westport)*. 1998; **38**(4): 289–96.

26 Rocheberg-Halton J. Emotions, things and places. In: Lupton D, editor. *The Emotional Self: a sociocultural exploration*. London: Sage; 1998.

27 This seems particularly significant as cleanliness and care are perceived as part of the mothering role.

28 Lovell A. Death at the beginning of life. In: Field D, Hockney J and Small N, editors. *Death, Gender and Ethnicity*. London: Routledge; 2001.

29 Mirren E, editor. *Our Children: coming to terms with the loss of a child*. London: Hodder & Stoughton; 1984.
Also, see Mirren's book for narrative accounts of loss, and the work of the compassionate friends.

30 Some of the women I interviewed directly refuted this.

31 See Deborah Lupton's work on the importance of possessions, used by women to represent themselves as 'mothers' in child-free spaces, such as work settings: Lupton D, editor. *The Emotional Self: a sociocultural exploration*. London: Sage; 1998.

32 See Carol Gitting's work for accounts of graveyard activities, including keeping animals and hanging out washing. Activities that might now be constructed as disrespectful but, at the time, maintained a connection between the worlds of the living and the dead.
Gittings C. *Death, Burial and the Individual in Early Modern England*. London: Croom Helm; 1984.
Also see:
Howarth G. Dismantling the boundaries between life and death. *Mortality*. 2000; **2**: 127–38.

33 There have also been accounts in the media and local newspapers, and local television news reports, of moves to re-formalise graveyards by banning or restricting the use of photographs and familiar terms (such

as 'Dad') on gravestones, and requiring parents not to put toys, balloons or windmills on child graves. These activities were seen by the authorities as disrespectful, whereas my research would tend to suggest that the personalisation of graves is important to mothers whose children have died. There are also media accounts of the removal of headstones away from the grave site to the perimeter of the graveyard to make the care of the cemetery easier – this, I feel, would be problematic for some grieving parents who feel that they are 'with' their child, when at the place of burial.

34 For an account of Tom Elder's feelings on visiting his daughter's grave see Pam Elder's account:
   Elder P. A portrait of family grief. In: Weston R, Martin P, Anderson Y, editors. *Loss and Bereavement: managing change*. London: Blackwell Scientific; 1998.

35 Also viewed by Wheeler as important following the death of a child and mentioned by Lupton as particularly evocative objects:
   Wheeler I. The role of linking objects in parental bereavement. *Omega (Westport)*. 1998; **38**(4): 289–96.

36 Diamond A. *A Gift from Sebastian*. London: Boxtree; 1995.

37 See Laakso and Pauhonen-Ilomen's work on mothers' experience of social support following the death of a child:
   Laakso H, Pauhonen-Ilomen M. Mothers' experience of social support following the death of a child. *J Clin Nurs*. 2001; **2**: 176–86.

38 Befrienders are lay people, who may have themselves experienced the loss of a child, who are associated with a support group and may offer to visit the newly bereaved to offer support.

39 To explore the differences between 'frontstage' and 'backstage work' see: Goffman E. *The Presentation of Self in Everyday Life*. Harmondsworth: Penguin; 1959.
   For consideration of the differences between public and private stories see:
   Ribbens J, Edwards R, editors. *Feminist Dilemmas in Qualitative Research: public knowledge and private lives*. London, Sage; 1998.

Chapter 3

The horror story of SIDS

The experience of SIDS can be configured as a love story in which the mother has to cope with the sudden loss of her child. However, this is only one of the stories about SIDS; there are other stories to be told. These are stories that may circulate at the same time and that interact with the love story. One of these 'other' stories is the horror story of SIDS. This is a version of SIDS that is often recounted in the media and has two main facets. One of these facets is the horror story concerned with the sudden death of an apparently healthy baby; the other is a particular narrative or story that circulated and was emphasised at the turn of the new millennium, in which SIDS deaths were scrutinised, and the inference made in some quarters was that some of these deaths at least were suspicious. One mother commented on her experience of the interface of these two stories:

'People say that the worst thing that can happen is for your baby to die – but the *very worst* is for someone to say, or to believe, that you killed them.'

Sudden and unanticipated death

SIDS is defined as 'the sudden death of a baby that is unexpected by history and in whom a thorough necropsy examination fails to demonstrate an adequate cause of death'. This definition has existed since it was suggested by Beckwith, an American pathologist, at the 1969 Seattle conference on sudden deaths in infants.

Since then, this basic definition has been adopted, with some minor modifications, as the basis for the World Health Organization classification of SIDS. Some discrepancies occur between the definitive explanations of SIDS in theory and practice in different countries.[1] This definition of SIDS relates to there being no known cause for the infant death. In other words, SIDS is what remains when the death has been investigated and no other cause has been found. Therefore it is a category of exclusion – other causes of death have been excluded. But there is still no particular cause of death identified. Hence the question may remain, 'Why did the baby die?' However, although a death cannot be classified as SIDS until after the pathology examinations have been completed, infants who die suddenly and unexpectedly without immediate identifiable cause will be considered as SIDS from the outset. Because no definitive cause of death is identified, there can be no ultimate sense of closure. As more information emerges about SIDS, the cause of death may be revisited. At one level this is about the advances in medical knowledge. But it also leaves scope for deaths to be reconsidered for other reasons. For example in some court cases,[2] the death of a second or subsequent child led to the re-consideration of the cause of death of the first child. This is distressing and problematic for parents whose children have died. The lack of closure and identification of a cause of death is difficult for parents who have a subsequent child, as they still do not know why their child died and therefore may feel they cannot adequately reduce the risk of a recurrence. There are schemes which support parents when they have another baby, such as the Care of the Next Infant programme (CONI).[3] However, these support systems often focus on additional surveillance of the infant, via use of apnoea monitors, temperature monitors and other measures, and this can be problematic in associating these activities with prevention.

Not knowing

One of the difficult issues associated with SIDS is not knowing what caused the baby's death. This can lead to a sense of guilt that the carer should have noticed some change in the baby's behaviour or appearance, even though there may have been none. This also may lead to a sense of guilt – that there must be a reason why the baby died. Sometimes mothers may worry that other people feel that they could have done something to prevent the death.[4] There is also the concern that if it is not known why a baby died, then another death could occur. Although the occurrence of two or more sudden infant deaths in a family is very rare, it is not unknown.

Some of the women I met during my research mentioned the importance to them of uncovering a cause of death. But for others, it seemed to be more important to focus on finding a way of coping with their immediate experience of grief. Maybe for some, SIDS is seen, if not a cause, at least as a way of categorising what had happened – some talked about their baby having died 'of SIDS'. The complexity of the situation, with its uncertainties and instabilities in the way the category is applied and defined, is part of the difficulty of finding a way to cope with this type of infant death.

For most of the women I talked to, the suddenness of the death was absolutely overwhelming – that there was no apparent indication that the infant was going to die, and therefore there was nothing these mothers could have done to prevent it. There was a real sense of injustice that this could happen without the opportunity to intervene. And the helplessness of finding the baby, and not being able to do anything to resuscitate the infant, was a recurrent theme. Not knowing why the baby had died, not knowing what to do – this is one of the horror stories of SIDS – suddenly being thrust into a scenario for which one is totally unprepared.

Media stories

There were stories circulating in the media relating to whether some deaths categorised as SIDS were due to unnatural causes. Part of this arose following publication of an article by Roy Meadow (1999) relating to 'unnatural deaths'.[5] One of the arguments put forward at the time was that most of the preventable deaths had been prevented, and therefore the remaining deaths must include a number of unnatural or suspicious deaths. This was also accompanied by a debate in the media as to whether SIDS was 'masking' unnatural deaths.

Michael Green (1999) was quoted as encouraging coroners to be more rigorous in the way they investigated sudden infant deaths.[6] This initiative had originated in Australia – and the media coverage encouraged the debate to emerge in the UK. The protocol was called 'Think Dirty' and encouraged coroners to consider all potential causes of death in cases of sudden unexplained infant death. The effect of this was to increase the focus on SIDS deaths in the UK. SIDS was in the news, with reports relating to the 'Think Dirty' initiative; a high profile was given to court cases in which mothers whose infants had died and been classified as SIDS were accused of having been involved in the deaths of their children.[7] One of these cases involved the use of statistical evidence (later proved at appeal to have been flawed) in which the likely incidence of multiple SIDS deaths in one family was significantly underestimated. This in turn led to an increased belief that SIDS deaths could be due to unnatural causes in families experiencing multiple deaths, but there was also an underlying perception that this could possibly be the case in other deaths classified as SIDS.[8]

Media stories also emerged relating to what mothers should know and do in relation to caring for their children. This included a plethora of information – including the advice to 'avoid risky behaviour such as falling asleep on the sofa with an infant'.[9] This construction of mothering as including the ability to avoid potentially unplanned activities such as falling asleep, put maternal care under increased scrutiny. These were stories in which women and mothers were being placed at the centre of a scrutiny of childcare practices. The story runs that mothers should know about the risk of SIDS and should be avoiding all 'risky behaviours' – even when the behaviours associated with 'risk' are diverse and include unplanned activities, such as falling asleep, or things which may be outside of the mother's control. This would seem to imply that SIDS is preventable – and yet the 'cause' of SIDS deaths remained elusive. These inconsistencies were difficult for mothers to negotiate; indeed many of the mothers I interviewed described BtoS in ways which led me to believe that they viewed compliance with the guidelines as 'preventing' SIDS. Indeed one mother described how she had followed all the guidelines and commented:

'I did everything I could for this (the death of her baby) not to happen.'

This highlights a difficulty for health professionals working with mothers and their babies: how to get the message across about risk reduction in relation to SIDS without inadvertently misleading mothers into believing that SIDS is preventable.

Total compliance with guidelines such as BtoS is notoriously difficult to achieve – as circumstances may constantly differ. For example, a carer may be very careful about maintaining the temperature of rooms at home, but may be unable to control this aspect in other venues, e.g. at the homes of relatives, or on holiday. Likewise they may be very careful about positioning their babies when putting them down to sleep, but might unintentionally fall asleep whilst holding their babies. This may lead mothers and other carers to blame themselves for inconsistencies in following risk reduction guidelines if their child dies. There is another difficulty too, in that some mothers may choose *not* to follow the guidelines. This is an interesting issue to consider. In the 1980s, mothers were advised to put their babies to sleep prone (on their fronts), as this was thought to encourage any fluids to drain away from the babies' airways. This was common practice for a number of years. The research on which BtoS was based, however, uncovered a relationship between sleep position and overheating – a risk factor in SIDS. Babies sleeping on their fronts have a greater tendency to overheat than those placed supine (on their backs). The advice on sleeping position moved through 180 degrees from putting babies to sleep prone, to putting them down to sleep supine. For many mothers (and grandmothers) a total reversal in advice was difficult to accommodate. At one of the groups I attended, some mothers remarked on how they had put their babies down to sleep prone because:

'That's what my mother did with me and I was okay.'

and

> '. . . because that is what I did with my older children – and they were fine.'

These mothers expressed how deeply this had affected them, in feeling that they should have followed the guidelines. One of these mothers also commented that she felt unable to talk to people about this aspect of her child's care in case they blamed her and yet she told me about it. This seemed to suggest that mothers need to be able to talk about the aspects of the child's death which troubled them, without feeling that others were judging them for the decisions they had made. This is one of the aspects of the horror story of SIDS, in that mothers are somehow silenced and prevented from receiving the support they need, by their perception that others may judge them for the decisions they have made or for inconsistencies relating to child care. Yet, in general terms, parenting is often associated with compromise, of uncertainty as to what is the best thing to do, of being offered solicited and unsolicited advice on all sorts of issues, and having to decide what course of action to take.

What if it happens again? How can I prevent it if I don't understand what happened?

One of the emerging themes in the stories I was told about the experience of SIDS was the concern that it might occur again if the couple went on to have another child. This may have been influenced at one point by the media coverage of women who had had more than one child die suddenly and unexpectedly, and were on trial on suspicion of having caused the death of one or both of their children. The concern that another child might die was linked for some mothers to the failure to find a reason or cause for the death. As one commented:

> 'How can I prevent it happening again, if I don't know why it happened?'

This was a real concern for some parents. The inability to allay the feeling that the cause might be 'genetic' or 'something I didn't do right'. The death of their child had led to the scrutiny of these mothers and the way they had looked after their children. This took the form of the initial investigation into why the infant had died, but also a self scrutiny as some questioned themselves:

> 'Did I miss anything? Was there something I could have done? I don't think I can ever be sure.'

The burden of these thoughts was almost tangible in some of the interviews. Even though they had been reassured that they were not implicated in any way in the death, some mothers still questioned themselves.[10]

One mother was troubled by the fact that her baby had died despite her best efforts to comply with the BtoS guidelines. She told me how she had been worried about the risk of infant death from the outset, and had carefully and consistently followed the advice she had been given. She commented:

> 'I did everything I could for this not to happen.'

It seemed particularly hard for her to come to terms with the fact that the BtoS guidelines were concerned with risk reduction and not with prevention as she had believed. This mother was one of only a few women I met who commented on their own personal fear of SIDS occurring before it happened to them. That is not to say that other mothers had not been worried, but they did not express it to me as a concern. There were also two mothers who commented on how they had previously associated SIDS with women unlike themselves. One stated:

> 'I always thought it happened to people who smoked heavily, not to people like me.'

The other commented on how:

> 'When I saw SIDS mothers in the news they always seemed different to me – I can remember reading about a mother whose baby had been found by the nanny – and I can remember thinking at the time that I would look after *my* baby myself.'

This contrast between their previously held beliefs about families who experienced SIDs and their own situation led to some parents questioning their previously held views. One woman I met also felt that her previous understanding of SIDS affected her impressions of how people viewed her following the death of her child:

> 'I used to think that there must have been something that they could have noticed . . . something they could have done . . . people must think that about me now . . . it haunts me that I used to think like that.'

Ordinary actions with extraordinary associations

One of the aspects in which the loss of a child to SIDS can be thought of as a horror story is the total unexpectedness of the death. Mothers referred to the ordinariness of the preceding days and sometimes even the hours before their baby's death. For example, one mother commented:

> 'It was on the day the bins are emptied, I can remember the sound of the bin lorry on the street and thinking that things don't happen like this.'

Another mother I met at a support group told me how her baby had died in the middle of the afternoon:

> 'They call it cot death, but he wasn't even in a cot – it wasn't even night time.'

She had been on the phone to a friend in the next room and had returned to find that her baby had died. She remarked:

> '. . . just so ordinary, just talking to a friend on the phone – and in the very next room . . . well, you know . . . .'

The fact that there had been no warning and that the death occurred so quickly, was very traumatic for this mother to recall. She found it difficult to put into words the events of that afternoon. Others commented on the weather:

> 'It was a beautiful crisp morning, the sun was streaming through the window.'

Again the emphasis was on the ordinariness of the day, even the pleasantness of the day up until the point when they found their baby had died. These juxtapositions with the extraordinariness of the day with the ordinariness of the day underline the suddenness of the death. They also underline the fact that any ordinary day can suddenly change for any mother of a young child – it is this aspect that may be very difficult for others to cope with, as it is a reminder of the fragility of life and the helplessness of the parents in being unable to resuscitate the child.

I was looking after him – do others blame me?

On occasion I heard mothers wonder aloud whether others blamed them for the death of the baby. This ranged from the wider comments, already mentioned, in which mothers wondered whether society somehow views SIDS as preventable or occurring as a result of poor care. This was a position that was underlined by comments made in the court cases taking place at the time, articles by Meadow and others that were referred to in the press, and to some extent the stereotypes highlighted in the government and national reports. The latter was commented on at a support event I attended, when a mother said:

> 'Who are these people in these reports, the young, poor, heavily smoking mother whose baby dies – it's not us, is it?'

She was keen to highlight the differences between the prevalent view of the family whose baby dies of SIDS and the parents she had met whose infants had died.

There was another place in which the anxiety of being blamed for the death was visible, and this was in the concern as to whether people they knew thought there was something they could have done to prevent the death. One mother stated:

> 'I look at them sometimes and wonder if they blame me, I know they don't . . . but I still wonder.'

Murphy (1990)[4] also comments on wondering whether her husband might feel that she is responsible for the death in some way.

They also mentioned this anxiety about blame in oblique references; for example, one mother said:

> 'I don't suppose I will be asked to baby-sit for friends.'

Another told me:

> 'Some people will think of me as jinxed.'

In contrast to these comments there were also positive statements such as:

'My friend asked me to hold the baby – I was even nervous of doing that . . . but I felt she was trusting me with *her* baby . . . sort of letting me know that she didn't think I had anything to do with my baby dying. I felt really touched.'

Another commented:

'You actually want to be with babies, your arms ache to cuddle a baby, but for all sorts of reasons it is the last thing other people want you to do.'

There were other telling comments too, such as:

'I represent the worst thing that can happen, and that makes me difficult to be around.'

And

'No-one wants to be reminded that their baby can die suddenly, and for my friends when I am there . . .'

Although her words tailed off, the message was clear.

These feelings of being a constant reminder to other young mothers of the fragility of life made some social contacts particularly difficult. Some women remarked that a significant number of their friends were people they had met through being parents – via parent-craft classes and mother and toddler groups. They told me of friends who were really supportive and caring, but they also told of being excluded from some groups:

'Other mothers feel awkward coming to see me. They think I wouldn't want to see their children, although I would actually.'

Others mentioned how people avoided them, partly through not knowing what to say:

> 'People don't know what to say, so it is easier to not have contact . . . and yet I need contact with people even when I am sad.'

Another mother commented:

> 'People who live nearby cross the street when they see me coming – I sort of know why – but it feels really uncomfortable.'

Responses also reflected different viewpoints, such as:

> 'I quite like being left alone.'

This was a reminder that although patterns of similarity might emerge in accounts of grief, there is always difference too.

Some women mentioned how they liked to talk about their babies or to talk about the events that had happened to them. They also highlighted the difficulties in doing this:

> 'I don't want to worry or frighten other people.'

Another said:

> 'I want to say something, but I know I will get upset and that would be embarrassing for them.'

It was notable that even in their extreme loss, many mothers described being aware of other people's feelings. It seems to me that at the time when women need support the most, social attitudes to bereavement can isolate women.

Blue lights – ambulances and squad cars

One of the images which emerged in my mind as I progressed with the research was the way in which there was a mixture of very public and private events associated with the baby's death. One of the clear pictures which emerged in many conversations was sending for the ambulance. People commented on the 'blue flashing lights' as the ambulance arrived. The arrival of an ambulance with all the flurry of activity that accompanies it effectively causes a private event to be suddenly placed in the public domain.[11] Some mothers commented on the way in which the arrival of the ambulance drew attention to the situation. One commented:

> 'I was aware of all of these people watching out of the windows when we got into the ambulance – some concerned and some just curious.'

Another mother mentioned during a group session:

> 'A moment before I hadn't been able to think of anywhere to go for help, and then suddenly I felt like I was surrounded by all these people – it was really odd – I didn't think anyone would be aware of what was going on and there they were, watching it all.'

The arrival of an ambulance causes a stir in a community, as does the arrival of a police car as part of the subsequent investigation into the infant's death. Not all of the women I interviewed mentioned the police investigation of the death, but for those that did it had been a significant experience in a number of ways. The association of the police with authority and with investigation for wrongdoing is strong. Engagement with the police may revisit the feelings of powerlessness and maybe even misplaced guilt that are attached to childhood memories of being confronted with authority or authoritarian figures. This was articulated well by one mother:

> 'The minute I saw the police car I felt guilty – I knew I hadn't done anything to be guilty about, but even so, that was how I felt. You know . . . you'd feel the same if the police pulled you over when you were out driving . . . you would think . . . what now?'

Another mother similarly felt:

> 'The police . . . why are the police involved? . . . I felt cold inside.'

The association of the police with the investigation of why the baby may have died effectively has the potential for criminalising the death. This may then be reinforced unintentionally by the actions of the police. One mother told me:

> 'They took the baby's bedclothes away for examination . . . I asked them not to, but they said tests had to be done . . . I asked for them back a number of times . . . it took ages before they came back to me . . . and then they didn't smell the same . . . but I wanted to keep everything and they wouldn't let me.'

There is another aspect of the investigation by police that was important enough for mothers to mention, and this related to how they felt other people viewed the visit from the police.

> 'They will say that there is no smoke without fire, the police have been here.'

And:

> 'All the papers are full of that solicitor's case (Sally Clark) and then here I am getting a visit from the police, they might put two and two together and make an odd number.'

She went on to say:

> 'I didn't want it to matter to me . . . but it did and I felt awkward going out, I am sure it wasn't an issue really – but I felt as though it was, and it was something else to have to cope with . . . the police were really nice. It wasn't them, it was . . . oh, you know what I mean, I can't find the words, and it was all happening all at once.'

Another described it as:

> '. . . not being in a state to argue – you just go along with the flow, you don't have the energy or resources to do anything else.'

Another mentioned:

> 'It seems no time at all before people are coming to talk to you with clipboards and forms . . . you just aren't ready for it; it is a job for them, but not for me.'

It seems that at a time when women are distressed and vulnerable there are multiple different sources of difficulty and stress, from stories in the media, to people's views, their own reflections on what has happened, and the investigation of the death, all of which have to be navigated simultaneously. Add to this the period of waiting, which incorporates different aspects of waiting – for the baby to be buried, for the results of the post mortem and coroner's inquiry, and there is indeed a horror story that surrounds SIDS – a story of being buffeted by one wave after another at a time when one's own identity and relationships may be shifting as people individually come to terms with what has happened.

Notes and references

1 See the Beckwith definition in Chapter 1. Also, the International Classification of Diseases (ICD) uses the category 'Sudden Infant Death Syndrome', but the Office for National Statistics (ONS) includes in the statistics deaths with dual entries on the death certificate. SUDI (sudden unexpected deaths in infancy) classifications do not necessarily correspond with the ICD classifications or the Beckwith definition (CESDI, 2000). Also, see:
Mitchell EA, Becroft DMP, Byard RW *et al.* Definition of the sudden infant death syndrome. Keep current definition. *BMJ.* 1994; **309**(6954): 607.
2 See the Sally Clark case.
3 The CONI programme is a national UK initiative established in 1988, using designated health visitors. The project identifies mothers whose infants have died of SIDS and who are pregnant. Supportive visits are offered during pregnancy, and the mothers are offered increased support from the health visitor service following the birth. The support takes the form of additional home visits, opportunities to weigh the baby more frequently on calibrated scales, apnoea monitors and the monitoring of ambient infant temperature. These interventions are based on data that suggest that babies who die of SIDS may lose weight prior to the death, and that overheating associated with infections may also be a contributory factor. The main benefit to parents is the increased contact with the health visitor service and the opportunity this offers to build confidence and to reassure parents.
4 See Sarah Murphy (1990) for her account of loss, expressing the feeling she felt that she had failed her husband, '*He had entrusted our baby to my care and she had died while in my care. I don't think that he ever blamed me for her death but I would have quite understood if he had done so and I can understand the feelings of any father who feels that his partner must have done something wrong or failed to notice some vital sign that all was not well with the baby.*'
Murphy S. *Coping with Cot Death.* London: Sheldon Press; 1990. p. 38.
5 Meadow R. Unnatural sudden infant death. *Arch Dis Child.* 1999; **80**: 7–14.

6 Green M. Pathologists must think dirty on baby deaths. <u>www.news.</u>
   <u>bbc.co.uk/1/hi/health/443010.stm</u> (accessed 7 November 2006).

7 The women at the centre of these court cases were eventually, after
   serving time in prison, released following appeal.

8 See Meadow's work on unnatural deaths:
   Meadow R. Unnatural sudden infant death. *Arch Dis Child.* 1999; **80:**
   7–14.

9 Media articles, e.g.
   Rumbelow H. Sleeping on a sofa with a baby is a risk. *The Times.* 1999;
   3 December.
   Murray I. Baby killers hidden by cot death cloak. *The Times.* 1999; 7
   January.

10 Sarah Murphy also commented on this sense of questioning and self
   scrutiny in her book on the experience of losing a child:
   Murphy S. *Coping with Cot Death.* London: Sheldon Press; 1990.

11 See Goffman for consideration of the divisions between 'public' and
   'private' and how individuals manage these boundaries.
   Goffman E. *The Presentation of Self in Everyday Life.* Harmondsworth:
   Penguin; 1959.

Chapter 4

Stories without words – the picture book

This book is primarily concerned with stories and the way in which people described the events that had happened to them. But there are also stories that can be told without words. This for me can be typified by the importance attached to objects. When I first began to talk to women whose babies had died of SIDS, I noticed objects, but these were secondary in some ways to the conversations or stories. And yet as time went on, the objects seemed to increase in their importance, as I realised the importance of objects both in conversation, and as tangible elements of a story that needed to be told. If conversation and reflection are the repository of stories, then objects can often be the receptacle of memories. SIDS affects infants at an early age, and so they may never have 'spoken' words, although they have communicated with those around them. It may be that in these circumstances, the stories without words become even more important than in other contexts. I have likened the stories without words to a picture book, and in this chapter I want to highlight a number of significant 'pictures' that tell their own stories.

As already mentioned, there are stories that centre on the objects kept at home and objects that relate to the infant's grave. There were also objects that were kept by mothers for different purposes – some told a story about the child's health and subsequent death; in some ways these were stories about infants' bodies and how they had been cared for and loved. Other objects were about the infant's social world and told stories about how they were valued by their families and others, and about shared experiences. The latter also included an element of archiving in order to tell the story of the baby's life to others.

The first set of 'pictures' or images in the picture book is of the objects that some mothers kept relating to the infant's care. These included a variety of items such as the baby's healthcare and weight records. These are items that most mothers possess and most would keep, as these are the NHS records of a child's development. I was more interested to find that some mothers had kept post mortem records relating to their babies. This to me seemed unusual at first, as the post mortem is a particularly unpleasant procedure. Yet as I talked with the mothers and as I looked at the documents they sometimes showed me, I realised that these documents were, in their own way, reassuring to these mothers, as although they did not uncover a cause of death, they did underline that the child had been well cared for. Sometimes mothers put this into words:

> 'Look what it says: "normal" heart and lungs . . . "normal" – they couldn't find anything wrong.'

This mother found this reassuring, as it confirmed to her that she had not overlooked or failed to notice something significant. Another mother commented:

> 'They still don't know why it happened, but they told me there was nothing I could have noticed.'

I was also shown records of infants' weights and their developmental records that had been kept by the mothers. SIDS is, by definition, sudden and unanticipated, yet there is some suggestion[1] that in some instances, retrospectively, parents might identify some minor changes in health or routine in the days prior to the death. This research contributed to the development of 'Babycheck',[2] a system of self surveillance for children, which encourages parents to contact a doctor if their child has a raised temperature, or minor infection. The difficulty is, of course, that the majority of children suffer from recurrent minor infections in infancy. CONI also works on the theory that minor physical changes may be significant and can be identified and managed. This seems to some parents to send a signal that there are elements of SIDS that are preventable; and yet it could be argued that the philosophy behind the interventions is shared with those of BtoS, which emphasises evidence-based practices centred on risk reduction approaches.

In addition to the parent-held records that relate to child development and are maintained in conjunction with the health visiting service, many parents also initiate and keep their own records of their child's development in the form of 'baby books'. This practice has a cultural element and parents often record their infant's 'milestones' – relating to the 'first time' their babies engaged in particular activities such as smiling, sitting unaided, babbling, speaking, walking and so on. These records are important in not only remembering the infant, but also in affirming the caring relationship between mother and infant. Baby books are a clear expression of a mother's focus on her child and the way in which they have noted in detail aspects of their infant's life. These mothers placed great importance on the medical and personal records of their infant's progress.

The second area of importance in keeping records was the objects that related to their infant's place in the wider social world. These sometimes included objects that had been gifts for the infant from people both within and outside the immediate family. These included objects such as christening and birth gifts, which affirmed the way the infant was acknowledged and valued by others. The mothers who showed me these types of objects were aware of who had bought the item and their relationship to the baby. Cards given to the baby and condolence cards were also important in emphasising the baby's wider identity in society. Part of the role of a mother is to present their infant to the world, and these objects were tangible reminders of the individual people who had known and valued the baby. In cases of bereavement later in life,[3] there is evidence that the bereaved retain the possessions of the deceased, and derive comfort from owning and using things that they valued or routinely used. In the case of death in infancy, these types of objects have not been chosen by the child, but chosen for or on behalf of the infant. Therefore there is a double appreciation of both the relationship the child had with the giver and the pleasure they had as recipient. Quite a few of the mothers I met had kept soft toys and items of clothes that the baby had owned. There is a parallel here with the practice of many mothers, who keep items belonging to their baby once they have progressed past infancy. The objects are associated with positive and happy memories.

Singularisation and personalisation

Many of the objects mothers keep are mass-produced items that are similar to many available on any high street. However, in the process of being owned by the infant they become singularised. This is a term used by Deborah Lupton (1998)[4] to describe the way that an object which is universal becomes personal. She uses the example of a pair of shoes to indicate the way in which once worn by the wearer, the shoes alter to accommodate that particular person's feet and therefore become individualised. In the case of an infant, the clothes or toys become singularised or personalised, either through a change in the object itself, as with a pair of shoes, or through association. Daniel Miller (1987) in his work on material objects, and Helga Ditmarr (1992) in her work on how individuals define themselves through objects they possess, refer to the importance of so-called 'aspirational' objects.[5,6] These are objects that aspire to a particular lifestyle. In the case of parents, most objects to some extent could be termed as aspirational, as the parents seek to give their child the 'best start' in life. Hence, objects that are kept may be a reminder of those aspirations and the desire and endeavour to do the best for the baby, as well as reminding them of the infant.

Another way in which objects are personalised is through the medium of photography. Sometimes objects were kept alongside pictures of the baby holding the toy or wearing the clothes. The juxtaposition of the object and the baby picture added poignancy to the keeping of the object.

Life stories

One of the issues that emerged in talking to mothers about the objects some of them had kept was the importance of keeping an 'archive' of the baby's life. This included photographs, objects, letters and documents. Sometimes mothers referred to this as a way of keeping the memory of the baby alive. For some this was important because they had other children, one mother commented:

> 'Sometimes we (indicating her toddler) sit down here and look through her things and talk about her and how much we love her.'

On other occasions it was clear that the mother was concerned to keep the memory alive for future children. One stated:

> 'I will need to be able to tell my other (as yet unborn) children about their brother and what he was like. He will always be part of our family, he will always be their older brother.'

This mother highlighted her role as the custodian of memories relating to the infant, and with a responsibility to affirm his place in the family. Different items from the objects to the photographs perform the work of recording and preserving memories of the infant's life. What ties this disparate array of objects together is that they all connect to telling the story of the baby's life and death. The objects are also part of the mother's biography, for her life story is inextricably woven with the infant's.

It is also important to consider how the telling of life stories might change over time. The women I interviewed for my research were recently bereaved, whilst some of the mothers I met in other circumstances had experienced SIDS months or even years earlier. I was aware in listening to mothers that sometimes the stories had a different emphasis. Mothers whose children had died recently talked more about the chronology and the detail of events. The telling of these stories, illustrated with objects and pictures, was often very detailed and I was aware that they, and I as the listener, were to some extent making sense of, and searching for meaning in, the events that had occurred. They also often spoke at length and in a very moving way about their love for their infants. This latter feature of the stories was still present in the accounts of those whose infants had died some time before, but for many the chronology of the period that they related to had in some ways shortened, and they focused more on the events following the death than those of the days leading up to it. This may be a feature of where and how the stories were told: some were as one-to-one interviews to a researcher, and others were told in larger gatherings to a group of people, some of whom had also experienced SIDS. However, it may also be to do with how, over time, stories become edited, not because the importance of the content has changed, but because the time other people devote to listening has altered – what remains could be viewed as a distilled life story, in which all the elements are still there, but in a more concentrated form.

Acquiring new objects

Occasionally mothers commented on buying objects for their baby after the death – one mother described buying a necklace and putting it on her daughter at the chapel of rest. Others described continuing to buy a particular product because of the associations with their baby. One mother I met described using baby talcum powder herself:

> '. . . because the smell is comforting.'

Another mentioned:

> '. . . using the same perfume I used when she was first born, because it is a link with my baby.'

Some mothers mentioned buying objects to take to the grave:

> 'I still buy things – I put them on the grave; last week we took up a blue bunny and put it on the grave – it seems more appropriate than flowers.'

Another said:

> 'I take things like those little windmill things (making a spinning gesture) to put on the grave.'

These objects, whether they are associated with smell or texture, tell their own story of a need to constantly reconnect with the positive experiences of mothering, and a personal demonstration of their link with their child. They are in their own ways tokens of motherhood.

Innese Wheeler (1998)[7] in her work with link objects – the items parents kept after a baby died to remind them of their infant – went on to explore how parents used these objects as part of their grief. She discovered that parents variously stroked, held, kissed and hugged objects. These actions are ways of linking with the baby or child, but they also illustrate a continuing relationship with the deceased and demonstrate an ongoing identity as mothers. Wheeler discovered that some objects were more important than others in facilitating aspects of remembering and grief, and, of these, photographs were uniquely powerful in evoking memories of the infant. Lupton (1998) cites Rocheberg-Halton[4] in claiming that photographs are one of the most evocative emotional objects and have a capacity to evoke a strong response.

Often the mothers I interviewed showed me pictures of their children, and some also had pictures of their babies on display in the home. On one occasion my attention was drawn to a picture of the family on the wall. As the mother explained that the picture included the baby who had died, she mentioned that the photograph had been taken following the death. The picture was tasteful and appeared similar to many other family group portraits that adorn the homes of parents: a picture of parents and an apparently sleeping child. Yet here was a portrait taken after the trauma of the death. The mother went on to explain that some people would find the picture distasteful for that reason, but that she valued it as it was the last picture to be taken of the family together.

There were other occasions when mothers showed me photographs of the infant taken after the death. Some were Polaroid pictures taken in the hospital; others had been taken by the parents themselves. There is some precedent for this practice, in that many maternity departments photograph stillborn children for the parents. There are also historical precedents, as at the time of the research, an exhibition of post-death photographs of children from Victorian times was touring the UK. And yet mothers were also describing to me the disapproval they received from others at displaying this type of photograph. Comments included:

> 'My friend said it was "creepy" having the picture on display, but actually it's a lovely picture.'

And:

> 'My mother asked me to put that photo in a drawer – I haven't, but I do move it when she visits.'

This made me wonder about the changing practices relating to photography, and also how social conventions were disapproving of something which for some bereaved mothers was so obviously helpful. As with many other issues, these mothers conveyed that they had found a way of navigating these difficulties, sometimes by simply not pointing out that the infant had died at the time the photograph was taken. Some mothers commented that they wished that they had more photographs taken when the infant was alive. It was also interesting to note that some of the pictures parents treasured and showed me were not necessarily technically good photographs, but those which captured the personality or characteristics of the child. Hence, some were not even a clear image, but were still important and precious – evoking memories of shared events and occasions, as well as just remembering the appearance of the infant.

Notes and references

1   See Emery (2000), and for work on changes prior to death noted retrospectively. Also see Blair *et al.* (2000), Gilbert *et al.* (1990), Hodgeman (1998), Ponsonby *et al.* (1993), Ponsonby *et al.* (1998), Taylor & Emery (1983).
Emery JL, Waite AJ. Debate on cot death. These deaths must be prevented without victimising parents. *BMJ*. 2000; **320**(7230): 310.
Blair PS, Fleming PJ, Leach CEA *et al.* A clinical comparison of SIDS and explained sudden infant deaths: how healthy and how normal. *Arch Dis Child*. 2000; **82**(2): 98–106.
Blair PS, Nadin P, Fleming PJ *et al.* Weight gain and sudden infant death syndrome: changes in weight z scores may identify infants at increased risk. *Arch Dis Child*. 2000; **82**(6): 462–9.
Gilbert RE, Fleming PJ, Azaz Y *et al.* Signs of illness preceding sudden unexpected death in infants. *BMJ*. 1990; **300**(6736): 1378.
Hodgeman JE. Apnoea of prematurity and risk for SIDS. *Pediatrics*. 1998; **102**(4): 969–71.
Ponsonby AL, Dwyer T, Gibbons LE *et al.* Factors potentiating the risk of sudden infant death syndrome associated with the prone position. *New Engl J Med*. 1993; **329**(6): 377–82.
Ponsonby AL, Dwyer T, Couper D *et al.* Association between the use of a quilt and sudden infant death syndrome: case–control study. *BMJ*. 1998; **316**(7126): 195–6.
Taylor EM, Emery JL. Family and community factors associated with infant deaths that might be preventable. *BMJ (Clin Res Ed)*. 1983; **287**(6396): 871–4.
2   See Babycheck information on FSID website www.sids.org.uk/fsid/ (accessed 18 September 2006). Babycheck aims to be used as a tool to identify potential risk and thereby offer guidance and reassurance to parents.
3   Parkes CM. *Bereavement*. London: Tavistock; 1996.
Moss MS, Moss SZ. Four siblings' perspective on a family death: a family focus. In: Hockey J, Katz J, Small N, editors. *Grief, Mourning and Death Ritual*. Buckingham: Open University Press; 2001.
See Mirren (1984) for accounts of and discussion of the objects originally owned and used by the deceased that become important to the bereaved following a death:

Mirren E, editor. *Our Children: coming to terms with the loss of a child*. London: Hodder & Stoughton; 1984.

4 Lupton D, editor. The Emotional Self: a sociocultural exploration. London: Sage; 1998.

5 Ditmarr H. *The Social Psychology of Material Possessions: to have is to be*. Hemel Hempstead: Harvester Wheatsheaf; 1992.

6 Miller D. *Material Culture and Mass Consumption*. Oxford: Blackwell; 1987.

7 Wheeler I. The role of linking objects in bereavement. *Omega*. 1998; **38**(4): 289-96.

Chapter 5

A collection of short stories

Tales of resistance

When a baby dies suddenly and unexpectedly, a range of investigations are undertaken to ascertain the cause. These investigations are triggered via the certification of death and the inability of the reporting officer, often the hospital doctor in Accident & Emergency, to state a specific cause of death. Establishing a cause of death involves pathological examinations, a post mortem, interviews with the parents or carers to ascertain the circumstances of death, and consultation with health practitioners who may have seen the infant in the days preceding the death. Hence the investigation involves a range of people and services including the police, the family doctor and other professionals such as pathologists.

Often the general practitioner (GP) will not only offer an insight into the baby's health and development to assist with these enquiries, but will also be a point of contact for the mother who has lost her child. Within Western society, the family doctor is a key point of contact for validation of illness, as well as the treatment of the sick. Furthermore, the current welfare system utilises GPs as the point at which absence from work can be legitimised via the diagnosis of an illness or condition that precludes the sufferer from the necessity of being involved in the workplace. So it is the doctor to whom people are encouraged turn to in times of crisis, and it is the doctor who is burdened with the need to offer an appropriate response. Most of the women I interviewed mentioned visiting or being visited by their doctors following the death of the baby. On occasion this was to discover more about the process of investigation and in particular the outcome of the laboratory tests. In other instances, the contact with the doctor was a focus for talking about their experiences and their reactions to the loss. Most of the mothers I conversed with were not working at the time of their infant's death, being either on maternity leave or having taken a decision not to work whilst their children were so young. In UK society, compassionate leave is often set by employment organisations at 3–7 days, after which the bereaved must take either unpaid or annual leave, or alternatively seek a medical certificate from the GP stating that they are not fit to work. This means that one cannot be off work for being sad, but only for a 'medicalised' condition relating to sadness or bereavement such as depression. I was surprised to find that this culture had an effect even on women who, for whatever reason, were not currently in work.

Hence, the mothers I interviewed described how they often found that when they visited the doctor their sadness and grief was translated into medical terms. One mother put this very succinctly:

> 'They say when you go to the doctors you have six minutes . . . it's not long to discuss heartbreak is it? Not long enough to describe the catastrophe which has hit your life and affects everything you do.'

This statement about the brevity of the medical consultation seemed to sum up the pervasive approach of biomedicine and the way it offers solutions or management of problems. She went on to describe how the interview was couched in almost entirely physical terms:

> 'They ask you about how you feel, how you are sleeping and so on . . . and then you get pills for all the bits and pieces you describe . . . pills to help you sleep, pills to stop you feeling so

> desperate and sad . . . only, pills won't help and I think we
> both know it.'

This mother describes so well, the way in which her grief is broken down into composite parts: the insomnia, the crying, the low metabolism and inability to engage with everyday tasks. Each is reviewed and 'treatment' is offered; and yet this 'treatment' is not holistic and doesn't engage the whole person. It doesn't really 'see' the grief – but only its effects. This mother was at pains to explain that the doctor was a nice person, a caring person, but still she managed to convey that biomedicine was not offering her what she needed. Her sentiments were also expressed by other mothers:

> 'They (the GP) want to do something for you . . . they want to help . . . so they do it the only way they know how, with tablets . . . maybe the suggestion of someone to talk to . . . a group.'

Implicit in this account is the belief that the GP is doing their best – but that what is being offered is not what is required. Another mother commented:

> 'I don't want to be anaesthetised from the pain of this – I need to live it – I can't explain . . . the pain keeps me connected, even though it is unbearable . . . how can I put it into words . . . well, there aren't the words.'

Again there is that contrast between the 'treatment' offered by biomedicine – to anaesthetise, to tranquillise, to take the 'pain' out of the situation – the tendency to treat grief like an illness and the reality of an untreatable sorrow.

I was very conscious in these interchanges of the responses of some of these women to the 'medicalisation' of their grief, in that they chose to resist it. This was not a resistance that was visible in the public space of the consulting room. They accepted the prescriptions offered to them. They told me of kind words and kind gestures on the part of their doctors. One even described feeling sorry for the doctor in having to deal with situations like this. They accepted that the GP had done the best they could. They described picking up the prescription from the chemist, but at the same time determining within themselves that the medication would not be taken. I was interested in some of the reasons that they gave as to why they would not take the medication but would accept the prescription. One mother felt that she had to be seen to be compliant:

> 'I don't want to draw attention to myself – I thought I would take the prescription and then do nothing with it. It's not just the doctor . . . other people will ask me, "Have you been to the doctor?" and "Did he give you something?" and it is easier to just say "yes" but then do my own thing.'

Other mothers described a feeling that they didn't want to be 'sedated' or 'treated' and that it was easier to appear to accept help and then make their own decisions. As one put it:

> 'You don't want all of that, but you are not strong enough to fight it, so you just go with the flow.'

However, 'going with the flow' didn't involve, for her, taking the medication. This was a resistance of a kind. The use of the medical model in relation to grief was resisted. It was resisted in the bathroom cabinet, in which the tablets and other medication came to reside untouched.

I was interested that these women told me their tales of resistance, but seemed to keep them from those involved directly in their care. One mother mentioned how it was a relief to tell someone, but at the same time didn't feel she wanted to engage with her GP. This is a key issue relating to the way in which as a society we deal with loss and grief. One mother commented on how often the help friends offered was couched in terms of 'treatment':

'They suggest that I should take some sort of herbal remedy or go somewhere to convalesce, but I am not ill . . . I am sad.'

This preoccupation with the physical body and its treatment seemed highly problematic for some women, as it forced a comparison between seeing grief as symptomatic, disordered and abnormal in the way that biomedicine sees diseased bodies; and another way of seeing grief, namely as unpleasant, devastating, diabolical – but also normal. I am not saying here that bereaved people should not accept medical help with the relief of some of the effects of their distressing experiences; such help may well be helpful and appropriate. Rather I am saying that the stories people tell of their grief are multiple and many, and sometimes they are viewed by other people as singular, as though they can be met with a single pattern of response. The medical response may not be as universally helpful as people might imagine it to be. As Jane Littlewood suggests:

'. . . the lack of a desire on the part of the bereaved to resolve their grief can be viewed by others as a "complicated" or "abnormal" expression of grief and yet one could argue that all grief is "complicated" anyway and that people need the support to make their own way through it.'[1]

The comments of the women who identified in their own experiences the tendency for professionals to describe grief in terms of ill health led me to question the social context in which those who are unable to function fully through sadness and distress are pushed towards categorising themselves as 'unwell'. The implication is that bereavement and grief in themselves are not sufficiently recognised and supported by the state system. There is also a tendency to articulate grief in particular ways, and those whose experiences differ are labelled as suffering from complicated or abnormal grief. There is an argument to be made about the 'medicalisation' of grief and sadness, and whether it should be more openly challenged.

Resolution of grief

There is an assumption in much of the grief literature,[2] which is often focused on the loss of a spouse or partner, that ultimately the bereaved find a resolution to their grief. For Freud this was achieved, albeit slowly and at personal cost, by detachment from the lost object and re-attachment to a new one. For Parkes (1972, 1986), the recovery is typified by an ability to 'move on' or 'pick up the pieces'. However, Littlewood (2001) highlights that the widows she researched were clear in stating that:

> 'They have no intention of either "resolving" their loss or giving up their attachment to their dead husband.'

Indeed the suggestion that 'resolution' might occur was a source of discontent. Likewise, Hallam, Hockey & Howarth (1999) outline the desirability for many bereaved people of maintaining a form of contact and certainly an identity that is entwined with their relationship with the dead person. This for me seems to capture some of the feelings I heard expressed by mothers in different settings. They saw themselves as mothers to the infant who had died, they would always be mothers, and the child they had lost would continue to be part of their family. This might include references to them in conversation, photographs of them in the home – but would also include helping other siblings (present or as yet unborn) to know about their brother or sister. This latter was expressed by one mother very clearly in the comment:

> 'I have to be responsible for letting my other (unborn) children get to know him and how much we loved him.'

She saw herself as the custodian of the family, the source of stories that needed to be told in the future, of having a responsibility to re-make her family complete in being the repository of stories that would affect their identity and sense of self.

It is in this context that considerations as to the way that grief is described and understood by professionals is important. If grief is understood as a process that can be resolved, a trajectory that is traversed, then resolution becomes an achievable end point. So to choose another journey, to reject that end point and state that you don't seek resolution is to stand out and identify oneself as 'different'. There are other points to consider here – firstly that if professionals view grief as a process with 'outcomes', then there becomes a particular way of 'doing grief'. Furthermore, to grieve in other ways is then viewed as experiencing 'complicated' or 'abnormal' grief.

'Doing it my own way'

The women I met throughout the duration of the research project were engaged in navigating their own way through the grief process. Although surrounded by assumptions, guidance and expectations surrounding how people mourn, they were able to use public and private spaces to find their own way through the experience. There were patterns that emerged in their comments that indicated that they seemed to find similar things constraining and to find relief, if not solace, in other activities. Hence, the 'treatment' of the 'symptoms' of grief seemed for many to overlook the emotional heartbreak that they were going through. Many also reported using objects in their grief in a way that enabled them to have some control over their expressions of grief. Some found attending self-help groups useful, but for others, the tendency to view all mothers who had experienced SIDS as sharing a similar trajectory was problematic.

I particularly noted the areas where they 'resisted', in one way or another, the popular versions of SIDS and grief. So, they resisted identifying themselves as SIDS mothers, by and large, in favour of labelling themselves, if they labelled themselves at all, as grieving mothers. They also demonstrated an awareness of the models of bereavement, but some also made remarks that highlighted the limitations of these models. For example, many bereavement models outline 'anger' and 'denial' as part of the process of loss and grief.[5] One mother, in describing how she felt, commented:

> 'I feel angry, I am at the anger stage – well, I suppose, it's not 'anger' really, but that is what you would call it.'

In other words she demonstrated an awareness of the so-called 'stages' of grief, and could identify in a limited way with being at a particular place in the process such models outline. However, as she draws attention to use of the word 'anger', she is also explaining succinctly that the language of the model doesn't adequately or accurately reflect on her position or the associated feelings that accompany it. Another mother remarked:

> 'I am not sure what stage I am at now.'

Again this is a reference to the trajectories of grief which are circulated in the media – and of which people are often aware, at least in part.

A further aspect of the social awareness of these grief trajectories for some mothers was the tendency for others to offer them not just support and guidance, but to verge on telling them what to do. One mother told me:

> 'I have lost count of the number of times people, sometimes virtual strangers, have told me, "you need to do this" or "of course you will feel like that". I feel you can't do what everybody else wants you to do – sometimes they are telling you different things anyway . . . so you have to do your own thing.'

Another woman commented:

'You are always being told things, often contradictory things – but you don't have the energy to fight it, you can just be carried along with it all.'

As already mentioned, some of the women I interviewed also resisted the 'medicalisation' of their grief. There were other instances, too, of doing things differently to the expectations placed on them. Hence, some mothers used and displayed photographs that were taken after the death even though others were sometimes uncomfortable with their display. Others encouraged their children and friends to engage with the grave in ways that differ from practices of the general pattern of visitors to cemeteries, such as encouraging play.

Here and now – the ongoing relationship

One of the areas that mothers commented on, which links indirectly to the general understandings of grief experience that circulate in the media and population, was to do with their understandings of what constituted 'abnormal' grief. One of the areas identified was to do with the experience of phenomena associated with grief. This included sensing the presence of the baby, hearing the baby cry, or seeing the baby in both familiar and unfamiliar places. For example, one mother commented on how she often sensed the presence of her baby. She mentioned how sometimes she felt as though the baby were in the room or the car with her. This is a phenomenon that is reported in literature as being associated with widows: some felt as though their partner were in the room with them[4] and one group reported experiences such as 'feeling the bed go down' with the weight of their partner. It could be that the bereaved are reliving a repetitive experience that was a natural part of their lives together, or it could be something else.

Some of the women I interviewed also mentioned how they 'heard the baby' from time to time. This ranged from:

'. . . waking in the night because I hear the baby crying'
to
'. . . hearing snuffling noises, as though he were still in the cot'
and
'I hear noises of her moving about, especially at night.'

Some mothers commented that they were reluctant to mention these experiences for fear that other people would think that they had 'gone mad' or 'lost the plot'. These concerns, that a part of their grief experience would be regarded by others as problematic, contributed to an inability to discuss some of the aspects of loss that they had to cope with. One mother linked these noises with the realisation of her loss:

'I wake up in the night, or sometimes in the morning, thinking that I have heard something, and then for a moment it is as though she hadn't died, and then I remember what has happened.'[5]

Other mothers reported 'seeing' their baby. One mother I met commented that when she went past the room where her baby had last been put down to sleep, she could see again the scene when she found her baby dead. This was a hugely distressing recollection and one that was difficult to avoid. But the comments made by other mothers did not relate to 'seeing again' the events of the time when they discovered their baby had died, but rather the phenomenon of seeing them, unexpectedly, in familiar and sometimes unfamiliar places. One mother commented:

'I sometimes look up and for a moment I can see her playing on the floor or, once, curled up on a chair.'

Another mother describing her loss in a group situation mentioned:

> 'I can be driving along and I look in the mirror and then, for just a second, I catch a glimpse of her in the back, asleep in the car seat.'

Just as mothers reported the suddenness of being 'ambushed' by the sight of one of their infant's possessions and feeling a surge of sadness and loss, so these 'sightings' of the baby caused a feeling of grief. Although these mothers also commented that in some ways it was also:

> '. . . strangely comforting, as if she will never have really gone.'

Certainly the women, who mentioned this phenomenon to me, did not find it disturbing or distressing in itself, but only that it reminded them of their loss. Nor did they feel it was a problem for them, but they were concerned that other people would feel that there was 'something wrong' or 'I wasn't coping.'

Some women reported 'seeing' the baby when out and about. However, this seemed to be more of a case of momentarily mistaking by a glance another infant for their own. One mother I met at a self help group commented:

> 'I was out in town and I thought I saw her in a pram, just out of the corner of my eye – I stopped and looked properly and it was a little girl the same age wearing the same anorak – it was a bit of a shock.'

A variant of singularisation[6] is taking place in this context, in that a coat available through chain stores becomes in the mother's eyes individualised, and therefore seeing the coat evokes a personal memory. Seeing the deceased is not uncommon in grief and is discussed by other researchers working in bereavement.[7]

Hearing the baby cry

Although some mothers reported having 'seen' their baby in the days after the death, others described the experience of hearing their baby. For some this was in the context of 'hearing' the baby during the night. One mother, whose infant had slept in a cot in her bedroom at night, reported waking and whilst half asleep:

> '. . . hearing the baby move about . . . you know snuffling and shuffling the bedclothes.'

She went on to reflect that she almost immediately became fully awake and recollected that her baby had died. Other mothers described being in the house and 'hearing the baby cry'. One commented:

> 'The impression of crying was loud enough to make me stop what I was doing and listen out.'

For some, this was an indication of how much they wanted the baby to cry out:

> 'I am listening for her, because I suppose that is so much what I want to hear.'

For others:

> 'The sound is so familiar that I still hear it.'

And one mother felt:

> 'I know it is easy to think that it is just "hearing things" but I do actually hear it, and it is as real as you are.'

Whatever the phenomenon of 'hearing' the baby might be – the mothers who mentioned it did not seem disturbed by these sounds and impressions, but instead described them as comforting.[8] As already mentioned, this awareness of the deceased, in this case the infant, signals an ongoing relationship with their baby. Apart from 'seeing' and 'hearing' the baby, there were other incidences of continued awareness of the infant.

Sensing a presence

In some cases, mothers described an awareness of their infant being 'with them' or sensing the infant's presence. Other writers have mentioned examples of this type of continued relationship with a dead relative, and descriptions of the phenomena include conversations with the deceased partner in which the widow might describe events and incidences to their husband, or may ask them for guidance and advice.[9] There are reports that such phenomena may also involve 'seeing' the deceased person, often sitting in a familiar place. Other women describe how they 'feel' the person with them, for example sensing the presence of the deceased. Other accounts include widows reporting the close physical presence of their deceased husband, including a sense of being touched by their partner.[10] Far from being troubling, these women found these experiences comforting and reassuring.

This is important in understanding how the bereaved person may have a different perspective on loss than is prevalent in society. In Western culture the dead are often viewed as 'other' to the living. They must be 'relocated' elsewhere, and there is an expectation that communication with the dead as part of everyday life is either abnormal or disturbing. Funeral practices are important in this relocation of the dead, and there is an expectation that following the funeral the bereaved should begin to accept that the relationship is ended and pick up the pieces of their lives. However, in practice, the bereaved may not relocate the dead in this way, but actually maintain a relationship with the deceased, viewing death as a disruption rather than a cessation of their relationship. This may be seen as problematic by others who do not want to acknowledge that the bereaved are continuing their relationship with the deceased. It may also lead to a situation, which some of the mothers I met described, in which they feel unable to talk about these phenomena to others, however personally comforting they might find them, for fear of being considered 'unusual' or worse. One woman commented:

> 'Other people might think I was losing the plot, or going mad, if I told them what I have just told you.'

It was this fear that others would fail to understand the significance of these experiences and couch them in terms of being 'abnormal' or as a sign of 'complicated grief' that seemed to be an important factor in keeping them hidden. It seemed to me, that at a time of extreme grief, some of the women I met were also having to negotiate others' wariness and concerns at some of the events that accompany loss. This in turn contributed to a sense of 'otherness' from people around them, and emphasised the loneliness and isolation of the grief experience.

I asked one mother if she felt able to talk to the doctor about these experiences. She replied:

> 'He's the last person I would tell, although he is a good doctor and I like him a lot, but he might think I wasn't able to look after my other children.'

The fear of being seen as: 'unable to look after my children' was a real source of anxiety and one which other mothers hinted at. They constantly reported concealing some of their more powerful experiences and feelings from those in authority, as part of a wider concern that they would be seen as 'not coping.' At one of the events I attended, I heard a mother express her concern that:

> 'They might take my other (children) from me if they knew how I felt sometimes.'

This anxiety might have been provoked by the court cases that were in the media at the time, in which some mothers whose children had died of SIDS, and who were later accused of being implicated in the death of these children, had been given limited access to their surviving children prior to being taken into custody.[11]

Some mothers described other phenomena that they associated with their grief; these included a state of anxiety that did not seem to be triggered by specific and particular events, for example:

> 'Sometimes I just feel anxious and I don't really know why.'

For others there was a reluctance to engage with others which led to anxiety, one mother I spoke to described how:

> 'I feel anxious when I hear the door bell or the phone rings, just for a moment . . . other times I just don't answer it, I don't feel able to.'

Whether this was associated with the need to be alone, or whether it was connected with the discomfort and social tension felt by other people in visiting and talking to a bereaved person, it was difficult to say. One mother I met, who had lost her child some years previously, described how, in the weeks following the death, she often had an urge to:

> 'Sit in a corner, upstairs, just literally out of the way of the world . . . or even wanting to go up into the loft – I have spoken to women since who have felt something similar during postnatal depression – it's a desire to disengage, but also wanting to be safe, I think. At the time I felt it was both unusual and not unusual, but I certainly didn't tell people how I felt.'

Her comments indicated many things about her experience: a sense of isolation, both physical and emotional, a feeling people wouldn't understand; and a feeling she was doing something, which in general circumstances was unusual, but somehow fitted her experiences. She went on to say:

> 'I can't recall how long that feeling lasted, but talking to you now, I can feel something of how I felt then – a strange mix of feelings that are difficult to put into words, but no less real for that.'

At an event I attended there was some discussion around the extent to which maternal grief affected individuals in the period immediately following the death. Mothers variously commented:

> 'I used to be quite outgoing, but I feel really quiet now, it is an effort to talk to people'
> and
> 'I just feel tired all the time; it is a sort of heaviness which just will not go away.'

Others remarked on a difficulty in focusing on things, while others commented on:

> '. . . a need to be on my own, but then liking the company of other people sometimes – I guess you could call it indecisiveness.'

It would seem that some of these responses at least are familiar to those who work with the bereaved.

Responding to phenomena

As already mentioned, the mothers describing these phenomena generally viewed them in very positive and reassuring terms. Some also commented on their own response and also their general response to the ongoing relationship with their infant. Some mothers reported talking to the infant, again a phenomenon following bereavement that is reported elsewhere:[12]

> 'I still tell him things, and particularly when I am looking at his things, or near his room.'

This mother was describing triggers that facilitated her conversations with her son. For other mothers, these triggers were associated with places:

> 'Sometimes I'll go somewhere and I will think – you would have loved this – I go on to tell them so.'

Another mother described going to familiar places:

> 'I walk through the park and I talk to her – tell her that I love her very much.'

The grave was a particular place where some mothers mentioned talking to their babies. One commented:

> 'I go to the grave to be with him.'

She went on to mention talking to the baby as she visited. Some mentioned that their conversations included their aspirations of what the infant's future would have been. One mother remarked that as she was tidying the grave she sometimes sang:

> 'I often sing a little lullaby might seem strange to other people but it feels okay to me.'

One mother I met commented that her ongoing relationship with her infant included a sense of continued development:

> 'I think of her as growing, as bigger now.'

This seemed to suggest that there is a difference in how mothers might view their continued relationship with their infant. For some, there is a continued relationship with the baby they lost, whilst for others there is the dynamic of change – they go to the grave to visit a child. It was apparent at some of the groups I attended that there is an element in which many mothers whose infants have died do think about the age their child would now be. I often heard remarks describing a baby in terms of how old they would be or what they would now be doing. For example:

> 'He would have been thirteen if he had lived and would have been choosing his options at high school next year.'

In this way, these children are a part of their mother's biography in terms of what happened in infancy, but are also a part of their current and contemporary stories of mothering, in which they still are able to find ways to represent their babies to others.

Maintaining difference – avoiding stereotypes

As I listened to the stories women were telling me about their experiences of loss and grief, I was aware of similarities in some of their accounts, but I was also aware of the differences. This is important as I am not claiming that all the women I spoke to whose infants had died expressed the feelings and experiences that I have outlined. There is a tangible difference between people's experiences, and I met women only for a very short period of time, relatively speaking. It is important not to stereotype or group together what is a significantly individual experience. I am also cautious of trying to stay true to the meaning as well as the words of the conversations of which I was a part. This is a responsibility that lies heavily upon me, and has troubled me at times, as I have sought to find a way to put these stories into words.

Notes and references

1 Littlewood J. Just an old fashioned love song or a 'harlequin romance'? Some experiences of widowhood. In: Hockey J, Katz J and Small N, editors. *Grief, Mourning and Death Ritual*. Buckingham: Open University Press; 2001.

2 See Parkes (1972), and for the complex range of grief reactions that he grouped into: numbness, pining, depression and recovery. See Kubler- Ross (1969) and her work on anticipatory grief for an account of the process of denial, anger, bargaining and resolution. Also, see Irrizary & Willard (1998), Riches & Dawson (1998), Klass *et al.* (1996), Ironside (1996), Lewis (1961), Oliver (1999) and Talbot (1999) for accounts of responses to grief.

Parkes CM. *Bereavement: studies of grief in adult life*. Harmondsworth: Penguin; 1972.

Kubler-Ross E. *On Death and Dying*. New York: Macmillan; 1969.

Irrizary C, Willard B. The grief of SIDS parents and their understanding of each other's responses. *Omega Journal of Death and Dying*. 1998; **38**(4): 313–23.

Riches G, Dawson P, editors. *An Intimate Loneliness*. Buckingham: Open University Press; 1998.

Ironside V. *You'll Get Over It: the rage of bereavement*. Harmondsworth: Penguin; 1996.

Klass D, Silverman PR, Nickman SL, editors. *Continuing Bonds: new understandings of grief*. Washington, DC: Taylor & Francis; 1996.

Lewis CS. *A Grief Observed*. London: Faber Paperbacks; 1961.

Oliver L. Effects of a child's death on the marital relationship. *Omega Journal of Death and Dying*. 1999; **39**(3): 197–227.

Talbot K. Mothers now childless: personal transformation after the death of an only child. *Omega Journal of Death and Dying*. 1999; **38**(3): 167–86.

3 See Kubler-Ross (1969), Parkes (1986), Bowlby (1961) for various models of grief. See also the summary of models and perspectives on theories of grief to be found in Hockey, Katz & Small (2001). Also, other bereavement texts: Dickenson & Johnson (1983), Archer (1999), Foote (1997) and Riches & Dawson (1998).

Kubler-Ross E. *On Death and Dying*. New York: Macmillan; 1969.

Parkes CM. *Bereavement: studies of grief in adult life*. 2nd ed. Harmondsworth: Penguin; 1986.

Bowlby J. Processes of mourning. *Int J Psychoanal*. 1961; **42**: 317–40.

Hockey J, Katz J, Small N, editors. *Grief, Mourning and Death Ritual*. Buckingham: Open University Press; 2001.

Dickenson D, Johnson M, editors. *Death, Dying and Bereavement*. London: Sage; 1993.

Archer J. *The Nature of Grief: the evolution and psychology of reactions to loss*. London: Routledge; 1999.

Foote J. Time to grieve. *Nurs Times*. 1997; **93**(49): 23–5.

4 Littlewood J. Just an old fashioned love song or a 'harlequin romance'? Some experiences of widowhood. In: Hockey J, Katz J, Small N, editors. *Grief, Mourning and Death Ritual*. Buckingham: Open University Press; 2001.

Hallam E, Hockey J, Howarth G, editors. *Beyond the Body: death and social identity*. London: Routledge; 1999.

5 A phenomenon also described by the widows in Littlewood's study: Littlewood J. Just an old fashioned love song or a 'harlequin romance'? Some experiences of widowhood. In: Hockey J, Katz J, Small N, editors. *Grief, Mourning and Death Ritual*. Buckingham: Open University Press; 2001.

6 See Deborah Lupton's work on singularisation in her book, which has also been outlined in a previous chapter.

Lupton D, editor. *The Emotional Self: a sociocultural exploration*. London: Sage; 1998.

7 For examples see Littlewood (2001) and Moss & Moss (2001), as well as Walter (1999) and Parkes (1986) for examples of 'sensing' the presence of the dead.

Littlewood J. Just an old fashioned love song or a 'harlequin romance'? Some experiences of widowhood. In: Hockey J, Katz J, Small N, editors. *Grief, Mourning and Death Ritual*. Buckingham: Open University Press; 2001.

Moss MS, Moss SZ. Four siblings' perspective on a family death: a family focus. In: Hockey J, Katz J, Small N, editors. *Grief, Mourning and Death Ritual*. Buckingham: Open University Press; 2001.

Walter T. *On Bereavement: the culture of grief*. Buckingham: Open University Press; 1999.

Parkes CM. *Bereavement: studies of grief in adult life*. 2nd ed. Harmondsworth: Penguin; 1986.

8 See Hallam, Hockey & Howarth (1999) for a discussion of phenomena that are thought by others to be troubling, but which the bereaved consider comforting.

Hallam E, Hockey J, Howarth G, editors. *Beyond the Body: death and social identity*. London: Routledge; 1999.

9 Littlewood J. Just an old fashioned love song or a 'harlequin romance'? Some experiences of widowhood. In: Hockey J, Katz J,

Small N, editors. *Grief, Mourning and Death Ritual*. Buckingham: Open University Press; 2001.

10 Hallam E, Hockey J, Howarth G, editors. *Beyond the Body: death and social identity*. London: Routledge; 1999.

Littlewood J. Just an old fashioned love song or a 'harlequin romance'? Some experiences of widowhood. In: Hockey J, Katz J, Small N, editors. *Grief, Mourning and Death Ritual*. Buckingham: Open University Press; 2001.

Parkes CM. *Bereavement: studies of grief in adult life*. Harmondsworth: Penguin; 1972.

11 For example the Angela Canning case.

12 Mirren E, editor. *Our Children: coming to terms with the loss of a child*. London: Hodder & Stoughton; 1984.

Also see Pam Elder writing about her family's response to the loss of her daughter:

Elder PA. Portrait of family grief. In: Weston R, Martin P, Anderson Y, editors. *Loss and Bereavement: Managing change*. London: Blackwell Scientific; 1998.

Chapter 6

Conclusion: the atlas of grief experience

I began this book using the analogy of a library of books and considering the experience of SIDS through the medium of different genres of literature. Having considered the love story, the horror story, picture books and the short stories about maternal grief, I want to conclude by reflecting on how grief might be represented, not as a model or a trajectory, but more as an atlas. In an atlas, the maps may be different, some of them reflecting the topography of the land, some reflecting the social geography. Some maps are close-ups of a small area, and some locate the region within a country or a continent. There are similarities and there are differences. There are elements of the same area seen in different ways and from different perspectives.[1]

In considering an atlas of maternal grief following SIDS, certain 'maps' could be identified as potentially useful in outlining some of the experiences that the mothers I talked to identified as important. These included physical elements of the maternal grief experience, the importance of objects in grief, the need to resist certain aspects of the responses of other people, and the co-existence of public and private narratives – stories that are not singular, but multiple and varied.

Arms that ache to hold a baby

Many times during the conversations I had with women whose babies had died of SIDS they referred to their loss in physical terms.

This varied from describing themselves as 'empty' or experiencing 'a terrible emptiness'. Whilst one woman described herself as 'feeling barren' and another as 'hollow', another felt 'desolate'. These physical descriptions were not limited to feelings linked to being bereft; mothers also articulated their experience of loss as:

'. . . being like a physical pain'
and
'. . . an ache that won't go away – I don't feel it ever will'.

For some women this pain was expressed in a sense of tangible longing; one mother described her feelings of loss, stating:

'My arms ache to hold my baby again.'

For another mother this longing was accompanied by feelings of restlessness, she commented:

'I just can't settle to anything.'

For others the feeling seemed to be harder to articulate. Some of the bereavement literature mentions the physical pain associated with grief, for example describing the experience as being like 'a pain in the throat'.[2]

There are also other descriptions which allude to physical aches and pains. As already mentioned, the longing to have and to hold a baby again, and reaffirm their motherhood, had led some women to become pregnant again, and others to be hoping for an early pregnancy. One mother alluded to how:

'Other people have said that it is too soon, but they don't know how this feels, every part of me longs to have this baby.'

Her remarks indicated that these women constantly had to navigate their way through the comments and opinions of other people. As one mother I met put it:

> 'Nobody made all these remarks the first time I was pregnant – but now they feel that they can comment on whether or not it is a good idea – not everyone of course, some people are really supportive and pleased for me, but I can see it in some people's faces that they think it is too soon.'

These descriptions highlight grieving bodies and the response of the women themselves and others around them to the physical manifestations of their loss and grief. Coping with their bereaved bodies also sometimes involved managing the suppression of lactation – which was described by some as a traumatic experience, as it accentuated their loss. Some also felt a physical need for another baby and were already pregnant or planning for another pregnancy. Alongside this was the awareness of the physical effects of grief including sorrow and crying, but also physical aching, insomnia, depression, lack of appetite. One mother commented on feeling continually 'nauseous' and another described an 'abdominal griping pain'; they also described 'pains in the chest' and 'headaches', restlessness and also 'a feeling of lethargy and fatigue . . . everything is an effort'.

If part of the atlas of grief is concerned with the physical aspects of loss and grief, then other parts of the atlas focus on managing to navigate the constant environmental reminders of their loss. They also commented on the (infrequent) occasions when they momentarily did not experience a sense of loss:

> 'I woke up last week, the sun was shining and just for a moment it was like stepping back in time – I felt happy – and then I remembered and the reality of what has happened came crashing back.'

Another mother commented:

'At times I can be waking up . . . you know the time when you are not awake, but you are not asleep . . . and just for a tiny moment – it is as if none of this had happened – then I feel almost guilty that even for a fraction of a second I could not remember . . . but at the same time . . . it makes me feel that it may be possible one day to . . . Well I don't know, there is somewhere I can move on to . . . .'[3]

Some of the comments made by the women I met indicated that the unanticipated exposure to an object associated with their infant, or a memory, was more difficult to cope with than anticipated ones. For example, coming across an object belonging to their baby, or relating to childcare, was particularly upsetting. Examples included being in a conversation that turned to a shared memory, or coming across one of the baby's possessions. For one mother this was the discovery of a half-opened packet of baby food in the cupboard; for another it was finding her baby's mitten under the sofa whilst cleaning. Other incidents they mentioned included the scent of particular flowers, or a specific brand of baby toiletries, or seeing another child in similar clothes to those worn by their own infant. This was in contrast to the way some mothers used objects in their grief as links with the baby, and as a way of purposefully recalling aspects of their relationship with the baby. Mothers often described how they liked to reminisce about their infants, either alone, or in the company of other people, even though this was sometimes upsetting. However, they also described being 'overtaken by grief' and how difficult this could be to manage. It was also highly significant to me as a listener, that much of the bereavement literature written for parents minimises the importance of objects in grief. Whilst keepsakes are mentioned, along with mementoes and sites for reminiscence and remembrance such as gardens, trees, benches, and so on – the importance of objects in maternal grief is often overlooked.[4] Objects associated with their infants were very important to the mothers I met. Those who had been bereaved for some years also described keeping multiple objects, and although they might not use them as frequently as they once did or in the same way, they had not lost any of their significance as link objects. I was also aware that for many practitioners, training focuses on the importance of relationships, conversation and companionship or even counselling following a loss – and yet in focusing on the human aspects of grief, the importance of the non-human elements – such as objects and places – can be completely overlooked. Objects seemed to play an important part in remembering their infant, but they were also significant in reaffirming maternal identity. Reminiscence involved recalling their mother–child relationship as well as the infant. This might have been one explanation for the diversity of objects some mothers kept, including clinical documents and paperwork, as well as photographs and toys.

Putting the record straight

In addition to the physical aspects of grief and the use of objects, there were also parts of the conversations I had with mothers which related to SIDS and their understanding of the stories circulating in the media. One of the things that had happened and been reported in the media at the time I was conducting some of my research was a legal case in which statistics had been used to calculate the probability of SIDS occurring twice in one family. The statistical evidence had been given by an expert witness who was a paediatrician, but not a statistician, and was later re-examined as there were errors in the calculation. One of the mothers I visited was particularly concerned by this statistical evidence. Her baby had died some time previously, but she was engaged in offering support to other women whose infants had died of SIDS. She explained to me how:

> 'I have looked on the internet and done some research to show that more than one death can occur in a family – I am able to tell people that the information in the papers is wrong.'

It was important to this mother to be able to correct what she understood to be misconceptions about SIDS. Another mother told me:

> 'People think that SIDS is an illness, I used to think that, but it isn't – and I tell people it isn't.'

Another mother commented on the government report into sudden deaths in infancy:

> 'It says in there that SIDS happens to young mothers who are smokers – that isn't me.'

This point was endorsed by a mother at a SIDS support group I attended:

> 'Who are these stereotypical mothers who are reported in the press – it certainly isn't us, is it?'[5]

In each of these cases, the women are demonstrating an active aspect of their grief in that they have become knowledgeable about the characteristics of SIDS. Their 'expertise' in knowing about SIDS leads them to challenge some of the misconceptions and misunderstandings about SIDS that appear in the media. This seemed to me to indicate another part of the atlas of grief surrounding SIDS, in that mothers develop specific knowledge and insights into SIDS and may become in themselves sources of information. Ultimately the knowledge they acquire is not just about grief and loss, but about SIDS itself, and they can be a powerful resource in challenging some of the stories which circulate around SIDS.

Public stories – I wouldn't want to worry them

I was aware when talking to women whose infants had died that there are mixtures of both public and private stories that co-exist around the experience of maternal grief following SIDS. I felt that sometimes I was permitted to be a witness to some of the private stories that mothers told, but certainly not to all. Erving Goffman describes the presentation of self in everyday life as involving both 'front stage' and 'backstage' work.[6] In other words there are some stories and activities that we present to the wider world and some that are hidden. This is a theme that is also explored by others,[7] along with a recognition that the social context may shape the stories we tell, and that some stories or 'voices' may be 'subdued' or 'silenced'. Sometimes the expectations that accompany mother-hood mean that mothers struggle to maintain a 'personal voice' as they internalise the expectations and perspectives of those around them. Jane Ribbens (1998), reflecting as a researcher on her own experiences of motherhood, comments:

> 'Over time I have come to realise that, even when I try to "listen" to my own voice and to "know" my own feelings and wants, other images and other voices intervene.'

She goes on to speak about her own 'voice', her own stories, being 'drowned out' by others. She further comments:

> 'It is not enough just to do the right things with my child; I am supposed to have the right feelings to go with the actions, and this is as central a part of motherhood as I have experienced it in this society at this period of time.'

It could be argued that these comments could be translated into grief experience too – in that individuals feel that there is a script that they are expected to follow, and that somehow in following it the nuances of their own stories and struggles can be somehow lost or hidden. The expectations of others may lead to 'feelings' being 'monitored, silenced or shaped.'[8] An argument is made that, referring to other research,[9] girls may learn during adolescence how to disconnect from their own knowledge and feelings in an attempt to connect with what other people want. In such ways women learn to present themselves in ways that are viewed as appropriate and acceptable to others and, in doing so, may conceal their feelings.

Some of the stories that women shared with me were ones that they felt might be unsuitable in some situations. For example, one mother described being with a friend who was pregnant:

> 'I feel inside that if SIDS could happen to me, then it really could happen to anyone – but I wouldn't say that to her, because I wouldn't want to worry her.'

This was an example of how, even at a time of personal sorrow and distress, mothers could have regard for the feelings of others. Another commented:

> 'When people ask me how I am, I usually say I am okay, because they are being polite and it wouldn't be right to say how I really feel – some people wouldn't know what to do and would be really embarrassed.'

This comment reflects the difference between the depths of conversations that women might have in different locations. It also reflects an awareness of a shifting personal identity, in that their grief becomes a factor in their relationships, and they may respond in ways that they feel are appropriate to the enquirer, rather than reflecting their own thoughts and emotions.

There is also a contrast between public stories and private stories in that some mothers reported that there were things that they found helpful and things that were not. Some mothers commented that friends tried not to mention their baby in their presence, yet as one said:

> 'I would like them to, and it wouldn't upset me too much.'

Another commented:

> 'I like it when they use his name – that's what the befrienders do, they always use his name.'

Some of the mothers described things that they kept hidden out of consideration for the feelings of other people:

> 'I can't talk about it to them; they wouldn't be able to cope'
> or
> 'Some things are just beyond words.'

Others kept things private for fear of the consequences, such as anxieties about their other children:

> 'People might think I am not coping.'

Others felt obliged to comply with other people's expectations:

> 'There is a feeling that you should be getting a little better all the time – but that is actually not how it is.'

One mother described her grief experience as:

> '. . . a dark tunnel, with no end in sight . . . and then one morning I heard the birds sing, and I thought, I haven't heard that for weeks, months even. I felt I was beginning to come out into the light, just a little bit.'

She went on to describe how she had been functioning 'almost normally on the outside, but just empty inside'.

Reflecting on mothering

On one occasion I spent some time with a group of parents whose infants had died of SIDS. One of the sessions was centred around their memories of their children – and people began to talk about the days preceding the baby's death. Some of the women there had quite recently lost their babies, and others had been bereaved for some time. They began to talk about the day their baby died and then the conversation turned to the day before the death; the final complete day that they had spent with their babies. They talked about how they treasured the memory of that day. They described the day, some in great detail, the little routine acts of mothering, the cuddles, the lullabies – their enjoyment in recalling their babies was almost tangible. They described what their babies were wearing, their toys, the things they had done together. And then one mother asked the others:

> 'If you had that day again, would you do anything differently?'

There was a bit of a pause and then it seemed to me that the mothers began to affirm that it had been a good day, an ordinary day in some ways, but totally unspoiled by what was to follow. One commented that she was glad she hadn't known what the future held as it had been a good day – my impression was of a halcyon day stored in her memory, alongside many other good memories. The consensus of the group, after some discussion, was that they wouldn't have changed things on that day with the benefit of hindsight; they had spent the day like many others loving and caring for their babies. These were memories of an ordinary day, which in itself expressed the extraordinariness of maternal love. It was a group conversation that had an effect on me, one I still revisit in my mind, in that it seemed to affirm the good things about motherhood and mothers. These were women who had subsequently travelled a difficult path, but could look back and remember taking the time to enjoy the early part of the journey.

Short stories

The stories I have told here are not, and could never be, the whole story. They are short stories. They are abbreviated versions of a big and ongoing narrative. They are mainly the stories which were told by women in the period immediately after their baby had died. Some were the accounts of women who had experienced SIDS months or even years ago, but these were in the minority. I listened to some stories in interviews and others in group settings. Many factors affect the way people tell their stories, if not the stories themselves. I noticed that in the group settings, women had found a way of telling their story in brief and relating it to the experiences of others. By contrast, the interviews were often quite detailed. Those who had told their stories many times had, it seemed to me, found a way of framing and shaping their stories, focusing on particular events and feelings. Their stories were meaningful and helpful to others. In a way, they had distilled the story into an essence – something that they could tell others in small compact spaces of time. I was keenly aware that this was a distillation and that their stories were much more complex and larger than this. In a way, this leads me back to where this book began – that we learn throughout our lives different ways of putting into words the things that happen to us, and in doing so we have to find beginnings and endings of sorts. But these are not finished stories, and even though the telling of them may become condensed, the story itself continues to grow. Many writers have commented that grief does not go away, but over time those who grieve find a way of living with, or in spite of, it.

One of the women I met had experienced SIDS many years previously – she described how:

'. . . finding my baby that day, shattered my life – nothing would ever, ever fit together in the same way again. But good things have happened since . . . I have had other children, whom I dearly love. So in a way, although the picture shattered, some of the bright fragments remain and others have joined them – like a kaleidoscope I have colour in my

> life, but also sadness – and the pieces make a pleasant picture, but I am always aware it is not the one it used to be.'

A final word . . .

During the process of my research, I learned a great deal. Sometimes I found the conversations upsetting, sometimes difficult, but always compelling. From the moment I met the first mother in my study and she began to tell me about her experiences and show me some of the objects that were so much a part of her grief, I was drawn into a new way of seeing maternal grief following SIDS. These are stories that I felt should be told, even if difficult to put into words. We are surrounded by stories, some of them are more important than others. We need to listen carefully. We need to hear. We are witnesses to the lives of others. We need to take note of the stories people tell about SIDS.

Notes and references

1   David Armstrong describes in his book how medical students are taught to relate to an atlas of the human body – explaining how organs relate to one another, and therefore study individual bodies alongside the 'atlas' to identify ill health. I am suggesting that grief experience could also be viewed in these terms – that there is a series of patterns, of ways of seeing grief, which can be useful in interpreting the experiences of individuals.
    Armstrong D. *Political Anatomy of the Body: medical knowledge in Britain in the twentieth century*. London: Cambridge University Press; 1983.
2   Parkes CM. *Bereavement: studies of grief in adult life*. 2nd ed. Harmondsworth: Penguin; 1986.
3   There are multiple accounts of the bereaved dreaming of their lost loved one and then realising on waking that the person had died; for examples of this type of phenomenon, see Parkes (1972) and Littlewood (2001).
    Parkes CM. *Bereavement: studies of grief in adult life*. Harmondsworth: Penguin; 1972.
    Littlewood J. Just an old fashioned love song or a 'harlequin romance'? Some experiences of widowhood. In: Hockey J, Katz J,

Small N, editors. *Grief, Mourning and Death Ritual.* Buckingham: Open University Press; 2001.

4 See Bradbury (2001), Francis *et al.* (2001) and Walter (1999) for examples.

Bradbury M. Forget me not: memorialization in cemeteries and crematoria. In: Hockey J, Katz J, Small N, editors. *Grief, Mourning and Death Ritual.* Buckingham: Open University Press; 2001.

Francis D, Kellaher L, Neophytou C. The Cemetery: the evidence of continuing bonds. In: Hockey J, Katz J, Small N, editors. *Grief, Mourning and Death Ritual.* Buckingham: Open University Press; 2001.

Walter T. *On Bereavement: the culture of grief.* Buckingham: Open University Press; 1999.

5 Such stereotypes may indeed be a product of epidemiological data, which tends to even out differences in population studies.

6 Goffman E. *The Presentation of Self in Everyday Life.* Harmondsworth: Penguin; 1959.

7 Ribbens J, Edwards R, editors. *Feminist Dilemmas in Qualitative Research.* London: Sage; 1998.

8 A further quote from Ribbens & Edwards:

Ribbens J, Edwards R, editors. *Feminist Dilemmas in Qualitative Research.* London: Sage; 1998.

9 See Brown and Gilligan (1992) cited in: Hearing my feeling voice? In: Ribbens J, Edwards R, editors. *Feminist Dilemmas in Qualitative Research.* London: Sage; 1998.